Extreme Health

Extreme Health

The Nutrition Connection

James H. Guest, DC, CCN

Copyright © 2002 by James H. Guest

All rights reserved. No part of this publication may be reproduced in any form or by any means, electronic or mechanical, including photocopy, recording, or any information storage and retrieval system now known or to be invented, without permission in writing from the author. For information contact drguest@drguest.com

The information in this book is not intended to replace professional medical advice. The author and publisher specifically disclaim any and all liability arising directly or indirectly from the use or application of any information contained in this book. This book contains my experiences and my opinions - not advice. Every individual has important differences in their physiological make-up. A health care professional should be consulted regarding your specific situation.

International Standard Book Number
1-59196-114-9

Printed in the United States of America
by
Instantpublisher.com

Contents

Introduction–The Mythematics of Science   7

Section 1 – Basic Building Blocks

Healing Is an Inside Job   13
What's So Complex About Carbs?   17
Protein   27
Fries, Lies & Heart Attacks   37
Nature's Food Processor   49
Gut Reaction   55

Section 2 – Some Thoughts on Disease Prevention

Disease: A Survival Mechanism?   63
A Bone of Contention   67
Nothing to Sneeze At   73
Is There a Doctor in the Joint?   79
The Heart of the Matter   87
Good Cells Gone Bad   97
The Dairy Dilemma   109
Going Against the Grain   119

Section 3 – Putting It All Together

```
Plant Power                    127
A Simple Plan                  131
Epilogue                       137
Recommended Resources          141
```

Introduction:
The Mythematics of Science

Many of us were taught in school that the scientific method is the "Gold Standard" of investigation and that it leaves no room for doubt. We are told almost daily that something has been "scientifically proven" or we hear the phrase, "scientific studies show…" and we tend to believe that it's true.

Problems arise, however, when we notice that some of these "scientific facts" seem to contradict each other.

A recent study says eating sugar does not change children's behavior. Another study found that sugar consumption raised adrenaline levels in children up to ten times normal. High adrenaline levels change behavior.

You read that a diet rich in beta-carotene will help protect from cancer and other degenerative diseases. Then you see a report that a group of smokers taking beta-carotene supplements actually had a higher incidence of lung cancer than smokers not taking the supplements.

A diet doctor says that carbohydrates should be severely restricted and that you can eat all the protein and fat you want. Another doctor believes carbohydrates should make up most of our diet and quotes studies that indicate vegetarians live longer than do people who eat meat.

What's going on here? We see all these 30-second "news" reports on television about some scientific discovery that contradicts what science told us a few weeks ago. Many people feel overwhelmed and confused. My goal is to clear up some of the mystery. I hope to "unwhelm" you a little.

Nutrition is a dynamic field. This book covers basic principles that are fairly stable, but nothing is absolute. Continue to read current articles and journals so you can keep up with new developments. Also remember that if you ask two nutritionists a question, you will probably get at least three different opinions. Don't be dismayed. Just realize that nutrition is part science and part art – and artists tend to look at the same things from different perspectives. This book is my attempt to bring you the basics of nutrition based on my knowledge, experience, and yes – my opinion.

Arthur Schopenhauer observed, *"Every man takes the limits of his own field of vision for the limits of the world."*

Arthur Koestler said, *"Every creative act involves ... a new innocence of perception, liberated from the cataract of accepted belief."*

Mark Twain said it simplest and best, *"Loyalty to a petrified opinion never yet broke a chain or freed a human soul."*

As you read this book, you may find that your beliefs are challenged. Please keep an open mind. The generally accepted "truths" of the past may be at least partly responsible for a significant increase in deaths and disability from a growing number of degenerative diseases.

A definition of insanity is doing the same thing over and over while expecting different results. How well have our current beliefs and behaviors served us? Why do half of us in the "developed" countries die from heart attacks and another 20 to 30 percent die from cancer? Why are so many of us disabled from arthritis, diabetes, and other degenerative diseases when these conditions are seen much less frequently in many other cultures?

If there is no room for improvement in your life, don't read this book. But if you want to become healthier and are willing to learn, read on.

Nothing in this book is intended as advice for any condition. For help concerning any health problems, please seek professional advice.

Section 1

Basic Building Blocks

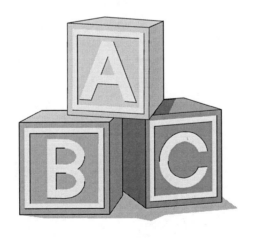

Chapter 1
Healing Is an Inside Job

When you cut a steak, does the wound heal? No? Let's help. After the meat is cut, sprinkle some vitamins into the wound. Add some wheat grass, barley grass, minerals, antibiotics, blue-green algae, fresh juice and herbs. Apply a few stitches to close the wound. Check on it a few weeks later. Will you find it nicely healed? Of course not.

Why do we heal, but a steak doesn't? It's because of something Hippocrates called "physis" – the life force present in all living things. The word "physician" comes from "physis." **True physicians strengthen the life force of the patient. Anything that interferes with this life force diminishes our capacity to heal.**

In his book *Health at the Crossroads*, Dean Black, Ph.D. says it this way: When we have a quart sized challenge and a pint sized capacity to handle the challenge, we can choose to reduce the size of the challenge or to develop a larger capacity. If we choose to increase our capacity, we not only handle the immediate challenge, we have also become stronger and better prepared to meet new challenges. In other words, we increase our physis – our life force.

For example, when we have an infection we can take an antibiotic to kill the bacteria (reduce the size of the challenge) or we can strengthen our immune system (increase our capacity). Sometimes antibiotics are necessary, but when improperly used, they actually impair the immune system.

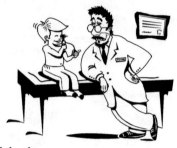

Research on ear infection illustrates this principle perfectly. According to the studies, children who were given antibiotics suffered recurrence more often than did children who were not given antibiotics.

The drug apparently lowered the number of bacteria so the challenge was smaller, but nothing was done to keep it from happening again (and again and again). Now we read about strains of bacteria that no antibiotic can kill, which probably developed because of overuse and inappropriate use of antibiotics. Ironically, the drugs have weakened us while strengthening the microbes.

Drugs and surgery are sometimes essential, but we often use them when safer options are available. When we use a hammer to kill a fly on our nose, we kill the fly, but pay a high price.

Before we can understand how to improve health, we need to know what optimal health is: **Optimal health is when all of our systems are working at peak efficiency.** No doctor, drug, supplement, surgery, therapy, adjustment, pill, powder, potion or lotion can heal you. Healing is an inside job.

To improve our health, we must do two things: Enhance our life force and remove interference.

Factors to be considered include our physical, environmental, emotional, and spiritual aspects. In this book, we will primarily limit ourselves to the nutritional components of our life force. You will discover that the **Standard American Diet (SAD)** is deficient in many elements essential for life force enhancement and it produces significant interference.

Chapter 2
What's So Complex About Carbs?

For centuries, alchemists have been trying to turn lead into gold. If they could just rearrange the components a little bit, something common could become something of great value. Plants – through the magic of photosynthesis – are masters of alchemy. Using energy from the sun, they change carbon dioxide and water into oxygen and a vital food called carbohydrate.

Carbon dioxide (CO_2) is a waste product of animal metabolism. We release it into the air every time we exhale. Water (H_2O) is vital to both plants and animals. A plant splits the carbon dioxide into carbon and oxygen. It releases the oxygen into the air for us to breathe and it saves the carbon.

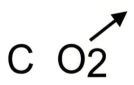

It splits the water into two parts (H and OH)

H OH

Then it combines the H's and OH's with the carbon. This simple rearrangement creates carbohydrate.

```
 H    H    H    H    H
 |    |    |    |    |
 C  - C  - C  - C  - C
 |    |    |    |    |
OH   OH   OH   OH   OH
```

The same building blocks become something with entirely different properties. The plant has converted a poison gas and a liquid into a solid, essential food, and gives us life-sustaining oxygen as a by-product. **Wow!**

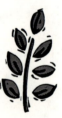

Big deal - so Mother Nature has a few tricks up her sleeve. What does that have to do with me?

The answer is simple. Without carbohydrate, you wouldn't be able to think, move, breathe, or even be alive. Thank you Mr. and Mrs. Plant. Our cells change carbohydrate into energy so we can run, jump, play, make love, see, speak, hear, and a few other things we tend to enjoy. The plant captures the sun's energy. We consume it. Our body uses it, then releases it back into the universe to be recycled. It is truly a beautiful system.

In addition to being a source of energy, carbohydrate is essential for the proper burning of fat. It is also used in many important structures such as DNA (the D stands for Deoxyribose – a sugar). In the form of fiber, carbohydrate binds with toxins and excess cholesterol in our digestive tract and carries them out of our system. Without enough carbohydrate in our diet, our body will begin to burn protein for fuel causing us to lose muscle and other important components.

Carbohydrate is also vital for the growth of beneficial bacteria that live in our intestines. These friendly critters manufacture several B vitamins, vitamin K, and help prevent yeast infections, parasite infestations, and more.

OK, Professor. Enough with the C's and O's and H's and OH's. Give me some stuff I can use in my daily life.

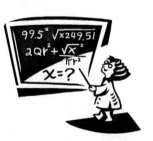

Fair enough. If you read magazines or watch television, you have heard about simple and complex carbohydrates. What's the difference? Why should you care?

Please forgive me, but I have to use a few more big words to answer these questions. Simple carbohydrates (sugars) come in basically two forms. Glucose, fructose (fruit sugar) and galactose are <u>monosaccharides.</u> When we combine them in pairs, we get the other form of simple sugars called <u>disaccharides.</u> For example when glucose and fructose are combined, we get sucrose (table sugar). When we put glucose and galactose together, we get lactose (milk sugar). Another example: Glucose + glucose = maltose (malt sugar). Don't worry, I'm not going to test you on this.

Complex carbohydrates are long chains of the carbohydrate units. They can be in the form of fiber, glycogen (the body's storage form of carbohydrate), dextrin, and starch. These long chains are called <u>polysaccharides</u>.

Does the structure really make any difference? Aren't they all carbohydrates?

I'm glad you asked. Suppose you need a new car. If you have the money, you just go buy one and drive away. This is like your cells saying they need some new sugar – a new car (*bohydrate*). If money (insulin) is available, the cells just pull it out of the blood.

On the other hand, what if the car dealer gives you a couple of truckloads of rocks, crude oil, plants, and sand. He is providing you with a complex car. All you have to do is extract metal from the rocks, turn the crude oil into plastic, create rubber and cloth from the plants and glass from the sand. Then you manufacture your engine, tires, body, transmission, seats, windshields, radio, instruments, etc. from those materials. See! It really is a car.

I think you will agree that it will take a little longer for you to be driving around in the second example. It works the same way with the sugar. When you eat simple sugar, your blood sugar rises very quickly. This causes a whole chain of events including the production and release of a hormone called insulin.

Insulin carries the sugar (fuel) into the cells and the blood sugar returns to normal. Sometimes the body doesn't react well to this sudden burst of sugar. It produces too much insulin for too long and causes the blood sugar to drop (hypoglycemia) or it doesn't produce enough insulin and/or the cells won't accept it so the blood sugar stays too high (hyperglycemia or diabetes).

Most of us can handle small amounts of simple sugars occasionally, but when we eat lots of these refined non-foods, we are asking for serious trouble. Simple sugar can increase triglycerides (fat) in our blood, increase obesity, cavities, suppress the immune system and much more. Although it can be burned for energy, it uses up nutrients that it doesn't provide so it "steals" them from our bodies. Many children eat more than their weight in sugar every year.

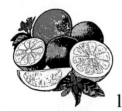

Fructose is a simple sugar that isn't quite as taxing because it can enter the cells without being chaperoned by insulin and therefore is less disruptive to blood sugar levels. **The best (only) way to eat fructose is in its natural state—in fresh fruit. Fresh, raw, ripe, organic fruit contains a wonderful combination of simple and**

complex carbohydrates along with lots of fiber and literally thousands of nutrients.

When we provide our body with complex carbohydrates, it has to break down those long chains into the monosaccharides and disaccharides (like getting metal out of the rocks) and this takes some time. Our blood sugar rises more slowly. The body responds carefully with the correct amount of insulin. The cells get energized and everybody is happy. In one study a group of college students lost an average of 18 pounds just by replacing sugar and white flour with complex carbohydrates.

OK, Doc. Quickly please! Where do we get these complex carbohydrates?

We get them from vegetables, fruit, and whole grains. You didn't think I could be that concise, did you? Well, you're right. I have to say a little more. The operative word here is "whole." Pasta, for example, is not usually made from whole grain. It is made from white (refined) flour.

The refining process removes most of the fiber and many essential nutrients. For many people, white bread acts pretty much like a refined sugar. Some people are so sensitive that they may have to reduce the amount of starchy foods like potatoes and even some whole grains.

Most of the "whole wheat" breads and rye breads, etc. that are sold in the supermarkets are really white bread with just a little bit of whole grain added for color and flavor. Read the label. If it says "enriched" flour, it is refined flour with a fraction of the lost nutrients put back in.

Fortunately, more markets and bakeries are providing true whole grain breads. Some are even made without added oil. These breads are heavier and it may take a little effort to train your taster, but after a while, you'll wonder how you ever liked the fluffy white stuff. Grains that contain gluten, however, may not be good for some people. See the chapter ***Going Against the Grain***.

In addition to having more vital nutrients, whole grains, fruits, and vegetables have fiber. In fact, dietary fiber is only found in plants. Plants are our friends, and they provide us with at least two types of fiber.

<u>Soluble</u> fiber can actually soak up excess cholesterol and toxins and carry them out of our bodies. Some of the soluble fibers – especially the gums such as pectin – can hold more than 50 times their weight. In addition to their janitorial duties, the soluble fibers and gums slow the absorption of carbohydrates resulting in better balance of blood sugar.

<u>Insoluble</u> fiber acts as a scrub brush for our intestines. When consumed with plenty of water, it can relieve constipation as well as reduce our risk of colon cancer, diverticulitis, and many other digestive problems.

Like other components of food, it is best to get fiber in the form of whole food, but it can be supplemented. Most of us should eat a <u>minimum</u> of 20 to 30 grams of fiber each day. Increase your consumption of fiber slowly. Work up to your optimal amount. Be sure to drink plenty of water when you increase fiber.

WARNING: A phenomenon called **insulin resistance** causes some people to have problems regulating their blood sugar when they eat starchy carbohydrates - even when they come from whole grain and potatoes.

Insulin normally binds to sugar and takes it into our cells where it is burned for energy. In some people, the cell receptors become resistant to the insulin. Even though the production of insulin is normal, it can't get sugar into the cells. The blood sugar remains high, so the pancreas produces even more insulin. This results in too much sugar and too much insulin in the blood in these resistant people.

Even though there is too much sugar in the blood, not enough is getting into the cell. So the cell says, "I'M HUNGRY – GET ME SOME SUGAR!"

We experience this as low energy and a craving for carbohydrate. We eat a cookie, or a sandwich, or a bowl of cereal, or some popcorn and guess what happens. The sugar still can't get into the cell very well so both blood sugar and insulin increase or at least remain at high levels and we are soon hungry again and want more carbohydrate. Some of you reading this will have experienced having a full stomach, yet still craving more food.

Things get even worse. Insulin not only escorts sugar into our cells, it is also involved in regulating how we burn fat. <u>When things are working right</u>, insulin slows fat burning, speeds sugar burning, and suppresses the appetite to bring blood sugar levels quickly back to normal. As soon as the blood sugar is where it should be, fat burning begins to increase.

However, if a person is insulin resistant, the resulting high insulin slows down the ability to burn fat, can't get sugar into the cells, and for some reason, doesn't suppress the appetite. So the resistant person stores the fat and still feels tired and hungry. As they store more fat (get fatter) they produce more insulin, get more resistant, become hungrier, eat, increase insulin, store fat...

It isn't lack of will power that makes them eat; it is a true physiological need for more fuel in their cellular furnaces. If this cycle continues long enough, in can develop into type II diabetes.

Insulin resistant people should totally eliminate refined carbohydrates (pasta, white bread, white flour, sugar, honey, etc.) from their diet and probably most starchy complex carbohydrates as well. This may mean avoiding all grains and grain products – even whole grains – and other starchy foods. And again, it's possible that others of us should avoid them too. (See **Going Against the Grain,** page 119)

Avoiding refined carbohydrates can:

- Decrease stress on your pancreas
- Lower the risk of diabetes
- Improve intestinal health
- Provide more nutrients
- Lower the risk of cardiovascular disease
- Decrease cavities
- Decrease obesity
- Decrease emotional disturbances related to extreme blood sugar highs and lows.

Chapter 3
Protein

Here is your chance to show off. Name the amino acids found in muscle.

Why can't you? You build new muscle tissue every day! How can you do that if you don't know the ingredients?

The point is, your body knows how to do lots of things that it doesn't tell you about. Chiropractors call this "Innate Intelligence". **Learn to listen to and trust your body – sometimes it knows more than you do.**

At any given moment, you are tearing down worn out structures and building new ones. You are also defending yourself against deadly attack, supervising thousands of chemical reactions, regulating your temperature and blood pressure, sending countless messages back and forth between your brain and body as well as between the cells themselves. One of the major materials that you use in accomplishing all this is protein.

Protein is made from building blocks called amino acids. Our bodies utilize 22 of these amino acids, but only eight are considered to be essential for most adults. This means that we must eat proteins containing sufficient amounts of the eight essential ones to remain healthy because our bodies are not able to manufacture them. We can build the others by breaking down protein, rearranging the amino acids, and putting them back together in a different pattern. Pretty cool. You didn't know you were so clever, did you?

Some of you will be disappointed and others relieved to learn that I am not going to list all of these amino acids for you. Most of you don't care and the others can go to the library or the Internet and look it up. I'll give you just a little more of the details, then we'll get into the fun stuff.

Remember carbohydrates? They are just atoms of carbon, hydrogen, and oxygen stuck together. If we add nitrogen and change the arrangement slightly, we have amino acids. All amino acids carry nitrogen. Some of them also contain sulfur, iron, or other elements.

We can't live without protein. Among other things we use protein for building muscle, bone, skin, hormones, enzymes, antibodies, energy, and more.

I could also tell you that protein is additionally involved in maintaining fluid balance, regulation of pH, synthesis of neurotransmitters, etc. I'm not going to tell you because then I'd have to write chapters on those things and tell you that pH stands for potential of hydrogen and explain all the intricate details of acidity and alkalinity and talk about acetyl choline and dopamine, but I'm too lazy to do all that. I will tell you the parts I think you need to know as we get to them.

One question that I'm often asked is "How much protein do we need?" The World Health Organization (WHO) says that consuming 4.5% of our daily calories as protein is plenty for good health. In fact, they say a generous safety factor is included in that number.

An article in the *New England Journal of Medicine* analyzed past and current research on protein requirements and presented the following recommendations.

    INFANTS 1.6g/kg/day
    AGE 10 - 12 .... 0.8g/kg/day
    ADULTS 0.5g/kg/day

What does this mean in Food? How does it translate to percentage of calories?

Good questions! I love your inquisitive mind.

I'll spare you the math, but it works out to 34 grams of protein per day for a 150 pound adult. This means that the entire daily protein requirement for this person can be satisfied by just 5 ounces of meat (½ a chicken breast, for example), or 2½ slices of a 15 inch cheese pizza, or 22 ounces of legumes such as beans and lentils. 34 grams of protein (136 calories) would be 5.4% of the total caloric intake for a person eating a typical diet of 2500 calories per day.

NOTE: While the protein in food is just 4 calories per gram, the fat it's packaged with may carry a lot of weight. For example the ½ chicken breast is 365 calories, the 2 ½ slices of pizza is 725 calories, but the 22 ounces of beans is only 150 calories. The legumes provide four times more food to fill you up (along with 25 grams of fiber and some complex carbohydrates), but only ½ to ¼ the calories.

So both the WHO and the scientists publishing in the *New England Journal of Medicine* seem to agree that around 5% protein is plenty. Now let's consult the real expert – nature.

Early infancy is a time of rapid construction, so we need a higher percentage of protein when we are babies than we do at any other time in our life. Notice that the *New England Journal of Medicine* study recommends about three times more protein for infants than for adults. I think most people will agree that the most perfectly designed food to support the rigors of infancy is the food that "nature" designed – human breast milk. The breast milk of women who nurture healthy babies derives 5% to 8% of its calories from protein. If that is enough for growing infants, then it is plenty for us grown-ups.

The average American eats about 15% of calories as protein – probably at least three times what we need. Even a vegan (a strict vegetarian who eats no animal products at all – no meat, fish, chicken, eggs, dairy, etc.) probably gets around 10% of their calories from protein because almost all vegetables and even some fruit contain at least that much protein. Beans and some other plants contain as much as 20 to 30% of calories as protein.

Is the protein in vegetables complete?

A few decades ago, a book called "*Diet for a Small Planet*" popularized some research that indicated vegetarians need to combine certain foods at every meal in order to get the right balance of amino acids. Two factors need to be considered, however. First, the research the book was based on concerned the dietary requirements of laboratory rats. Secondly, more recent research has discovered that we have an amino acid pool that will fill in the gaps if a meal is low in some amino acid. We do need to eat a wide variety of foods, but we don't have to eat them all at the same time.

Plant proteins are lower than animal proteins in an amino acid called methionine. That may be a good thing. Even though methionine is essential, too much can be harmful. The body converts it to a chemical named homocysteine, which has been linked to coronary artery disease and osteoporosis. Read more about homocysteine in the chapter **Bone of Contention**, page 61.

William Castelli, M.D., the director of the famed Framingham Heart Study, sums it up for us:

"Some people scoff at vegetarians, but they have a fraction of our heart attack rate and they have only 40% of our cancer rate. On the average they outlive other men by about 6 years."

Do athletes need more protein?

There is some controversy here, but it primarily depends on what you mean by "need". Yes, an athlete involved in intense training – not weekend softball – may need more than the 5%, but remember that most of us already eat three times that much. So the average diet provides more than enough protein for an athlete to stay healthy.

Frankly, many athletes are more concerned with performance than health. They want to know whether or not protein supplementation will increase performance. Depending on the sport, the answer may be "yes". For example, when Russian power lifters were fed about three times their normal amount of protein, they became stronger. Anabolic steroids also make people stronger, but damage their health.

Diets high in animal products increase our blood levels of an anabolic hormone called Insulin-like Growth Factor (IGF). While this hormone may be part of the reason muscle mass increased in the Russian power lifters, the long-term consequences of elevated levels has not been adequately explored. Based on the effects of similar chemicals, I believe the consequences may be unpleasant. Read more about IGF in my chapter, *The Dairy Dilemma*.

What is your opinion on the diets that recommend lots of protein and very little carbohydrate?

When you read the books that recommend restriction of carbohydrate and increased dietary protein, it sounds very scientific. There is another side to the story. I will end this chapter by citing some research that strongly suggests another point of view.

These protein promoting programs do help people lose weight and can lower cholesterol, but please consider the following information. **Cholesterol is not the only marker of heart disease. Others include homocysteine, lipoprotein-a, lipid peroxidation, fibrinogen, excess iron, and more.** Eating more meat and less vegetables and fruit may increase some of these factors. For example, a study published in the *American Journal of Clinical Nutrition* (October, 1978) found that "the risk of fatal coronary heart disease among non-vegetarian Seventh-Day Adventist males, ages 35 to 64, is three times greater than {that for} vegetarian Seventh-Day Adventist males of comparable age."

What about bone loss?

A study in the ***Journal of the American Dietetic Association*** compared the loss of bone density in lacto-ovo (dairy and egg-eating) vegetarian women from age 50 to 59 with omnivorous women (including meat in the diet) over the same period. The vegetarians lost 18% of their bone density while the omnivores lost 35%. Other research indicates that women who eat no animal products at all (vegan) lose even less bone than the lacto-ovo vegetarians.

What about cancer?

The International Journal of Cancer (September 1995) published a study of 25,892 women. This research concluded that the women who ate meat more than five times a week had an almost two and a half times greater risk of developing breast cancer than women who ate meat twice or less than twice a week.

The ***Journal of the National Cancer Institute*** (October 1993) printed a study examining the relationship between meat consumption and prostate cancer. The abstract states, "CONCLUSION: The results support the hypothesis that animal fat, especially fat from red meat, is associated with an elevated risk of advanced prostate cancer. IMPLICATIONS: These findings support recommendations to lower intake of meat to reduce the risk of prostate cancer."

What diet is best for diabetics?

In 1995, *Lancet* published research demonstrating that when adult-onset diabetics adopt a low fat, plant based diet, 75% of them are able to stop all medication. In another study, (*Postgraduate Medicine*, 1958), Dr. Walter Kempner at Duke University put diabetic patients on a diet high in complex carbohydrates. Within three months, most patients on his diet experienced a significant decrease in blood pressure, blood sugar, weight, insulin requirements, cholesterol, sugar in the urine, and protein in the urine. Since then, many confirming studies have been reported in the *American Journal of Clinical Nutrition, British Medical Journal, Diabetes Care, Lancet*, and others.

Other studies generate additional concerns:

A *British Medical Journal* study indicates a direct relationship between the amount of animal products consumed and the incidence of gallstones.

The *British Journal of Urology* reported that higher meat consumption correlates with more kidney stones.

Research published in the *Journal of Asthma* found that over 90% of asthmatics following a diet without any meat or dairy products could reduce or completely eliminate their medication.

A 1981 study in *Lancet* showed that vegetarian women had much less pesticide in their breast milk than the national average.

Another study in *Lancet* in 1991 reported that animal protein and animal fat aggravated arthritis symptoms while

100% of the patients on a strict vegetarian diet enjoyed significant improvement.

Vegetables, fruit, legumes, and whole grains provide literally thousands of protective nutrients. We are all biochemically unique and may need to adapt our food intake to meet our individual metabolic requirements. But at a time when most researchers are advising we increase our consumption of these healthy foods, we may want to be cautious of diets that restrict them.

Chapter 4
Fries, Lies & Heart Attacks

The word "fat" usually causes emotional reaction. To some of us gravitationally challenged people, it may bring feelings of guilt, isolation, self-condemnation, etc. On the other hand, the term "chewing the fat" means a pleasant conversation with a friend and "cream rises to the top" suggests that the fat is the best part of the milk. By the way, it recently occurred to me that within another generation or two, nobody will know what that expression means because nobody will have seen non-homogenized milk.

Is fat good or bad for me?

You've probably heard that animal fat is saturated and is bad for your heart and that polyunsaturated fat from corn oil and other plants is good for your heart. You may have also heard that olive oil is a monounsaturated fat. Let's explore what these terms mean and how these fats influence our health.

Saturated fat means the fat is saturated with hydrogen. This makes the fat very stable. It is normally solid at room temperature (and at body temperature) and doesn't react readily with other elements such as oxygen.

Unsaturated fat contains one (monounsaturated) or more (polyunsaturated) double bonds. A double bond is a relatively unstable connection between atoms. A hydrogen atom can attach itself at the double bond, so unsaturated fat is fat that is not saturated with hydrogen. Heat, light and oxygen can easily damage unsaturated fat. Saturated fats are the most stable and the monounsaturated fats are more stable than polyunsaturated fats. **Heating any unsaturated oil to cooking temperature is likely to damage the oil and produce free radicals.**

Any of the fats and oils we use contain a combination of different fatty acids (the building blocks of fats), but one type of fatty acid usually predominates. For example, saturated fatty acids are the major components of dairy fat, lard, beef fat and other animal fats as well as coconut oil and palm kernel oil. Monounsaturated fatty acid is the primary component of olive oil and peanut oil. Avocados also contain monounsaturated oil. Polyunsaturated fatty acids are the main building blocks of corn oil, safflower oil, flax oil, soybean oil, and many more.

We've been told that the polyunsaturated oils are good for us.

They can be very good for us if they are not damaged, but there is some conflicting information. For example, when it was discovered that consuming polyunsaturated fats lowered cholesterol, a study was undertaken that was expected to also show a reduction in deaths from heart attack. Two groups of people were put on the same low-fat diet. One of the groups consumed an additional four tablespoons of corn oil each day. As expected, cholesterol was lowered in the corn oil group. But surprisingly, the corn oil group had more heart attacks. Why? In my opinion, it was due to oxidation and the way our fats and oils are processed.

When you buy a bottle of cooking oil, it has probably been through the following steps before it was put in the bottle: The seeds are cleaned and hulled, pre-heated with steam, pressed in a high volume press that reaches temperatures of around 185 degrees Fahrenheit, exposed to a chemical solvent and more steam, distilled, exposed to caustic soda, refined, bleached, and deodorized at temperatures up to 520 degrees Fahrenheit.

The oil is then bottled in clear plastic and placed on shelves exposed to the fluorescent lights of the market. In other words, the oil has been severely altered before we buy it. I believe this is why the corn oil in the above study caused more heart attacks. The exposure to heat, light and oxygen creates free radicals. **Free radicals damage our cells - even our DNA.**

Are cold pressed oils better?

Not necessarily. "Cold Pressed" on a label usually means no outside heat was applied. The temperature of the press itself, and therefore the oil, can get pretty hot. You must choose a brand that takes care to protect the nutritional value of the oil.

Let's talk about why these oils are so important.

We previously learned that the building blocks for protein are called amino acids and some of them are essential – meaning our bodies must have them, but can't make them. It is essential that we eat them. Oils are similar. The building blocks are called fatty acids and two of them are considered essential. Linoleic acid is the essential omega-6 fatty acid. It is found primarily in corn oil, safflower oil, etc. Alpha-linolenic acid is the essential omega-3 fatty acid and is found primarily in green leafy vegetables, flaxseed, walnuts, and fish.

These two essential fatty acids follow separate pathways. Both lead to the formation of several hormone-like substances called eicosanoids. The omega-6 fats can lead to inflammatory or anti-inflammatory eicosanoids. The omega-3 fats lead only to the anti-inflammatory ones. For centuries, humans have consumed approximately equal amounts of omega-6 and omega-3 oils. For the last 100 years or so, food processing has increased the omega-6 and decreased the omega-3 until the **S**tandard **A**merican **D**iet has become quite out of balance.

How are good organic oils processed?

Certified organic seeds are cleaned and hulled then pressed in small batches at low temperatures in the absence of light and oxygen. That's it!

The oil is then put in opaque bottles – still with no light or oxygen – and immediately refrigerated. These oils are fresh and healthy. If you don't use them rapidly enough after they are opened, they start to become oxidized. You can smell and taste the difference. This doesn't usually happen because these oils are sold in small bottles.

<u>These are not cooking oils.</u> Whenever you heat polyunsaturated oils, you damage them. Use these oils in salad dressings, smoothies, or drizzle them over raw foods or other foods after cooking. **Keep in mind that any oil that has been separated from its source is concentrated and, in a sense, refined. Don't overuse them.**

What about olive oil?

Olive oil primarily consists of oleic acid – an omega-9 fatty acid. It is not an essential fatty acid, but it does have some advantages. When exposed to heat, light and oxygen, olive oil is much more stable than polyunsaturated fats (but less stable than saturated fats such as in coconut oil). Studies of people living near the Mediterranean Sea find that they have relatively healthy hearts and arteries, even though their fat intake (largely from olive oil) is around 40% of their calories.

It isn't clear whether this apparent protection comes from the oil, the phytochemicals in the olive, or some other factor such as the intake of fresh vegetables and fruit. Just remember that all fats – including olive oil – provide more than twice the calories per gram of carbohydrates and proteins. If controlling your weight is a problem, even olive oil can be overused.

The interactions and effects of these fatty acids are far too complex to address in a book intended to simplify nutrition. Those of you who want more detailed information can dig into any recent biochemistry text where you can enjoy the adventures of dihomogammalinolenic acid and learn about prostaglandins, leukotrienes and thromboxanes. Or you may prefer to read some of the more user-friendly books in my reference section such as **Turn Off the Fat Genes**, **Fats That Heal - Fats That Kill**, and **MegaHealth**.

What about fish oil?

In general, I consider plant oil to be healthier than animal fat if they are not damaged. Where do fish get their omega-3 oils? They get them from eating sea plants or by eating smaller fish that eat sea plants. Notice that fish do not heat or bleach or deodorize their oils. They eat oils in their most natural state. So should we. We should eat the plants that contain the oils. **In other words, we should eat whole food**. Plants that contain fat also contain fat digesting enzymes, fat-soluble anti-oxidants, and other protective factors. When we squeeze oils out of those plants – even good oils – we are isolating and concentrating them in a way that may not fit our physiology.

We may make some salad dressing using a bit of quality flaxseed oil, or maybe use a little olive oil to sauté something. But the best way to get our fats is by eating a wide variety of whole foods including vegetables, fruit, nuts, seeds, and grains. We also need to stop eating all of the processed and fried foods that contain huge amounts of the damaged fats that damage us.

If you choose to supplement with polyunsaturated fats, be sure to increase your intake of antioxidants. Fats oxidize inside your body and this oxidation can lead to long-term health problems.

What about Coconut Oil?

The coconut oil story deserves a special section of this chapter. In fact, many articles, papers, and even books have been written about this fascinating substance.

Coconut oil (composed primarily of saturated fatty acids) was widely used in commercial baked goods, and many other products for many years and then it fell into disfavor when it was publicized that saturated fats raise cholesterol.

I was taught that tropical oils such as coconut oil and palm oil should be avoided because of their artery clogging properties. More recently, a group called the Center for Science in the Public Interest (CSPI) conducted a mostly successful campaign to stop movie theaters from using coconut oil for popping popcorn. At first, I accepted all this at face value, but new knowledge has encouraged me to take a closer look.

Is coconut oil saturated? Yes.
Do saturated fats raise cholesterol? Sometimes.
Then we should avoid all saturated fats, right? No.
Is an increase in serum cholesterol always bad? No.

Now I've done it! Now I have to explain all those seemingly contradictory things. I've opened a can of worms and now have to fish or cut bait. (What else can you do with a can of worms?) Did that fill your cliché basket for the day?

First, let me acknowledge Mary Enig, Ph.D. As I began to research coconut oil, I discovered that Dr. Enig had already compiled what I was looking for. She has written many scientific papers and has given many lectures on this topic. A web search using her name will provide you with considerable detail on the information I'm going to summarize for you.

Some of the early animal research on coconut oil clearly indicated that consumption of it increases cholesterol. The word spread quickly that coconut oil was bad. There is a problem with this conclusion, however. Those scientists used hydrogenated coconut oil. This process adds trans fats. In other words, the results of the studies using hydrogenated coconut oil had nothing to do with natural coconut oil.

Animal studies using *unaltered* coconut oil found that it lowered the "bad" cholesterol and raised the "good" cholesterol. In fact, six times more cholesterol was accumulated in the tissues of animals fed polyunsaturated (and processed) safflower oil compared to the animals fed pure coconut oil. What a difference it makes when you use real food.

Human studies with coconut oil are very interesting. Studies of islanders with a high consumption of coconut found no adverse effects, but total cholesterol and LDL **increased** and HDL (the good stuff) **decreased** in those who **reduced** their coconut oil consumption.

Several studies indicate that when coconut oil is fed to people with high cholesterol, the cholesterol decreases or at worst, stays the same. When fed to people with normal cholesterol, the levels may go up a little, but it is from the

<u>HDL increasing while the LDL goes down.</u> That is a very good thing.

So, does coconut oil cause heart attacks? I believe it is very unlikely. It lowers bad cholesterol, raises good cholesterol, and "…animals fed regular coconut oil have less cholesterol deposited in their livers and other parts of their bodies". (Enig)

Why does coconut oil act differently than other saturated fats?

The other saturated fats and the polyunsaturated fats we talked about previously are long-chain fatty acids (18 or more carbons). The fatty acids that make up coconut oil are medium-chain fatty acids (12-14 carbons). This difference in structure makes a tremendous difference in function. For example, saturated animal fat is solid at body temperature, but the saturated fat from coconut is liquid at body temperature. Another example is that these medium-chain fats are readily used for energy and less likely to be stored as body fat.

There is a fatty acid in human breast milk called lauric acid. The baby drinks the milk and its body converts the lauric acid into something called monolaurin. Monolaurin prevents breast fed infants from getting most infections. Studies show monolaurin can inactivate bacteria, yeast, fungi, and viruses that have lipid envelopes such as the measles virus, HIV, herpes simplex, cytomegalovirus and others.

Why – you may ask – am I suddenly talking about breast milk in a section about coconut oil? It's because **the**

same lauric acid that protects breast-fed infants is the primary fatty acid in coconuts. When we eat coconuts and coconut oil, our bodies convert the lauric acid to monolaurin just like babies do and the monolaurin helps protect us.

Several studies in the 1980's indicate that coconut oil may also protect against cancer. Groups of animals consuming different diets were given chemicals that induce tumors. In one study, 32% of the corn oil fed animals developed adenocarcinomas in the colon. Only 3% of the coconut oil fed animals developed these tumors. Olive oil also seemed to protect the colon with only 3% developing colon tumors. But when the small intestines were examined, it was found that 7% of the animals fed olive oil had small intestine tumors and 0% of the animals consuming coconut oil had them. (For you non-scientists, that means none.)

The only way we can reap the benefits of monolaurin is if we consume lauric acid and lauric acid consumption has dramatically decreased over the past 40 years or so. We have been eating much more hydrogenated and polyunsaturated oils and less coconut and palm oils.

Dr. Enig points out that our population used to consume heavy cream and high fat milk. These are also sources of lauric acid. We used lots of dried coconut in cakes, cookies and pies as well as using coconut oil in many commercially baked goods. As mentioned before, movie popcorn was popped in coconut oil. Coconut oil was even an important source of fat in infant formulas. Now most of these sources of lauric acid have been drastically reduced or eliminated due to either misunderstanding or intentional misdirection.

It is my opinion that the saturated fats from coconut and coconut products are good for us. There is strong evidence that they protect against pathogenic microbes, and some tumors. They are quite possibly cardioprotective. Compared to the polyunsaturated fats, they are far less easily damaged by light, heat, or oxygen, which means they don't produce free radicals when used in cooking. I think they make a good addition to the diet.

Whew! This has been quite a chapter. I may have told you more than you wanted to know, but the information is valuable. Is what I have written carved in stone? Nope. Research and the amazing experiment called life will continue to alter our knowledge. What a fascinating life it is.

Chapter 5
Nature's Food Processor

Although the workings of the digestive system can be very complex, its basic purpose is simple: Let good stuff in and keep bad stuff out. You might think that swallowing lets stuff in – both good and bad – but that isn't really true.

Look at a donut. Suppose you hold the donut in one hand while you drop a penny through the hole. As the penny passes through the hole, is it inside the donut? Of course not. It simply falls through the hole without effecting the donut's structure, taste, edibility, etc. Our digestive system is basically a long, convoluted hole (tube) running from one end of us to the other. We could swallow that penny and unless it got stuck, it would "fall" through the tube and come out the other end. But this is a very smart tube. Let's take a quick tour.

One function of the digestive system is to break food down into very small parts — like a super food processor. Our biological food processor has mechanical blades called teeth that chop the food into small enough pieces to go through the tube. It also has chemical blades called digestive enzymes that chop the food into molecules that can be absorbed and utilized by our bodies. The enzymes chop proteins into amino acids, fats and oils into fatty acids, and complex carbohydrates (polysaccharides) into simple sugars (monosaccharides).

The first digestive enzyme is in the mouth. It is called salivary amylase and it begins breaking down carbohydrates as we chew. When food is well blended with saliva and enzymes, it is called a bolus. This bolus is pushed to the back of the mouth where it triggers a swallowing reflex. As it passes through the throat, a small amount of lipase — a fat digesting enzyme — is added to the bolus. The food makes its way through the esophagus to the stomach (and beyond) by muscular contraction called peristalsis.

In the stomach, the bolus is introduced to more chemical blades. One important chemical is hydrochloric acid (HCl). This acid is essential in helping enzymes such as pepsin, trypsin, and chymotrypsin chop up protein. It also tells the pancreas to release other digestive enzymes. In addition, hydrochloric acid is a valuable part of the immune system. It kills many undesirable bacteria and other teeny critters that find their way into our mouths and might otherwise make us sick.

The mixture of food, enzymes, and acid, is now called chyme. As the chyme leaves the stomach, the digestive system's next job begins – absorption. The architecture of the digestive system is incredible. Its surface area is about the size of a tennis court. Most nutrients are absorbed in the small intestine and specific nutrients are absorbed in specific areas. For example, calcium, magnesium, and most other minerals as well as fat, fat-soluble vitamins, and monosaccharides are absorbed in the first part of the small intestine called the duodenum.

Since it has just left the stomach, chyme is quite acidic and that is important. Calcium (especially calcium carbonate) cannot be absorbed efficiently unless it is in an acid environment. In my opinion, it doesn't make any sense to use an antacid as a source of calcium. There are better ways to handle indigestion and to get calcium. You can probably see how using the acid blockers that are so heavily advertised could disrupt normal digestion and absorption.

The second part of the small intestine is the jejunum. Before the chyme gets here, pancreatic enzymes and bicarbonate are added to continue the chopping process and to decrease the acidity. Disaccharides, water-soluble vitamins, and amino acids (proteins) are absorbed in this section.

Now the chyme moves into the ileum -- the third and last part of the small intestine where cholesterol, vitamin B12, and bile salts are absorbed.

The chyme then leaves the small intestine and enters the large intestine where water is absorbed, along with a few more nutrients. The large intestine is also the home of many helpful bacteria such as strains of acidophilus and bifidus. These friendly folks manufacture vitamins including B12, K, and folic acid. They also help prevent overgrowth of fungus, yeast, parasites, and other troublesome organisms.

Unfortunately, antibiotics kill good bacteria along with the bad, but they don't kill the yeast, parasites, etc. This imbalance is called dysbiosis and can lead to major problems. We will talk more about dysbiosis later.

As the chyme loses water in the large intestine it becomes feces. This is what's left after the body takes all the nutrients it can. It consists of bacteria, fiber, cholesterol, toxins, water, and whatever else the body rejected or was unable to absorb. The feces then pass out of our bodies and into a convenient toxic waste dump.

One critical factor in maintaining good health is complete digestion. If you are not fully digesting your food, it can lead to poor absorption and/or absorption of large, undigested molecules. **Digestive problems have been linked to fatigue, allergy, asthma, arthritis, malnutrition, cancer, heart disease, and more.**

Completeness of digestion depends on a healthy digestive system. The food must move through at a proper rate. Too fast — nutrients won't be absorbed. Too slow — foods will ferment and putrefy creating toxins that are absorbed into our blood.

The condition of the intestinal wall is also important. All the little hills and valleys that provide surface area can become smooth and decrease our absorption. Or the walls can become "leaky" and allow large, partially undigested molecules to get into the blood. This has been associated with food allergies and aggravation of chronic conditions such as arthritis. For more information, see the chapter on allergy: *Nothing to Sneeze At* (page 73).

Why is digestion and absorption so important? **Every component of your body – every cell, tissue, organ, nerve, chemical, etc. – comes from what you eat.** Your cells regenerate constantly and the only building material available comes from our food. This makes our food choices incredibly important. Do we want to build our house out of straw, sand, or rock? It appears that some of us want to build our house out of soft drinks and hamburger. According to Eric Schlosser's book *Fast Food Nation,* Americans drink about fifty-six gallons of soft drinks per person each year. Some drink less and some drink a lot more. About 20% of children one or two years old now consume soft drinks. He also states that in addition to the soft drinks, Americans now eat approximately three hamburgers and four orders of French fries every week. If we truly are what we eat, our cells are in big trouble.

In my opinion, addressing any health condition or disease without evaluating and enhancing the digestive system is providing less than optimal care. Unfortunately, most health care professionals have not been adequately trained in this important area.

For a more comprehensive look at digestion, I recommend you read *Digestive Wellness* by Elizabeth Lipski. It is easy to read and provides a wealth of great information

Chapter 6
Gut Reaction

As I mentioned in the Digestion chapter, our intestinal system is in a sense, outside the body and has two major functions: to let good stuff in and keep bad stuff out. It lets good stuff in by absorption and by a process called active transport that requires carrier molecules, receptors and gets complicated. It keeps bad stuff out by acting as a barrier and by activating the immune system against anything that gets through the barrier that shouldn't.

Inflammation can disrupt all of these functions. When inflamed, the gut lets some bad things in and keeps some good things out. Active transport quits working well and the barrier function is much less efficient. Large undigested or poorly digested molecules – macromolecules – can "leak" through the gut wall into the blood stream. Common causes of gut inflammation include bacterial infection, viral infection, parasites, alcohol, many anti-inflammatory drugs, food allergens, lactose intolerance, caffeine, refined carbohydrates, and more. It's easy to understand that most of us have a system that is at least a little bit leaky.

So what?

I'm glad you asked. When these macromolecules get through the wall, antibodies are formed that may contribute to rheumatoid arthritis, multiple sclerosis, lupus, allergies, and many other conditions. Bacteria and candida in the digestive tract can get into the bloodstream. The carrier proteins involved in active transport are damaged leading to nutrient deficiencies. IgA – an immune component – is reduced and we are left more susceptible to infection. Digestion and absorption are reduced. More free radicals are produced. Reactive by-products may damage cells in the liver, bile ducts, and pancreas. Just to give you an idea of how big a problem it is, here are some research titles:

Gastrointestinal absorption of unaltered proteins in normal infants
Pediatrics

Elimination diet and intestinal permeability in atopic eczema: a preliminary study
Clin Exp Allerg

Increased intestinal sugar permeability after challenge in children with cow's milk allergy or intolerance
Allergy

Intestinal permeability in pediatric gastroenterology
Scand J gastroenterl

The leaky gut of alcoholism: possible route of entry for toxic compounds
Lancet

Effect of non-steroidal anti-inflammatory drugs and prostaglandins on the permeability of the human intestine
Gut

Aging-associated increase in the intestinal absorption of macromolecules
Gerontology

A short review of the relationship between intestinal permeability and inflammatory joint disease
Clin Exper Rheum

Abnormal bowel permeability in ankylosing spondylitis and rheumatoid arthritis
J Rheum

Most people with any type of inflammatory problem, allergy, intestinal disease, arthritis, or other chronic condition will have at least some degree of excess permeability. There is an intestinal permeability test for those who want to know for sure. It involves drinking a liquid that contains two non-digestible carbohydrates. One consists of large molecules that cannot move across a healthy intestinal wall. The other has smaller molecules that can get across, but have to have help – called active transport – that only a healthy gut can provide. Then by checking what shows up in the urine, we can tell what's getting across the intestinal wall and what isn't.

How do you fix a leaky gut?

A general approach to this and many other gastrointestinal problems has been described by Jeffrey Bland, Ph.D. as the "4R" program. Dr. Bland is a biochemist who has been studying and teaching nutrition for many years.

The first step is to **Remove** any thing that might be irritating the system. These things may include dietary irritants such as coffee, alcohol, food allergens, etc. It might also be necessary to test for and remove any harmful microorganisms or parasites. There are tests to identify these critters and to find out which remedy is likely to be the most effective.

The second step is to **Replace** any thing that is present in a healthy system, but is missing or low in an unhealthy one. Items such as digestive enzymes, intrinsic factor, and hydrochloric acid fall into this category.

Third, we **Repopulate** the intestines with healthy "friendly" bacteria such as acidophilus, bifidus, and others that are essential to keep the "bad guys" from getting the upper hand. These critters also synthesize some important nutrients.

Finally, we provide the nutrients needed to **Repair** whatever damage has been done. These items may include vitamins, minerals, amino acids, bioflavonoids, and antioxidants, to name a few.

Inflammation of the gastrointestinal system can let bad stuff such as toxins, allergens, and bacteria get through the wall and into the blood stream. It can also keep good stuff out such as the nutrients needed to build and repair everything in your body. Kind of important to fix it, don't you think? Returning good function to the digestive system has helped people with such diverse conditions as chronic fatigue syndrome, fibromyalgia, irritable bowel syndrome, food allergies, chemical sensitivities, skin problems, gastritis, and many, many more.

The only source of raw materials our cells, tissues, and organs have to rebuild and repair themselves is the food we eat. A faulty digestive system can truly impair <u>everything</u> else. An experienced nutritionist can help you identify and fix many digestive and intestinal problems and in turn, allow your body to function better and heal itself.

Section 2

Some Thoughts and Research on the Prevention of Disease

Chapter 7
Disease: A Survival Mechanism?

Disease is an amazing mechanism for survival. Don't be dismayed when you have a cold or the flu. The fever, sweating, coughing, nausea, diarrhea, runny nose, etc. are all working to get rid of the organism that has chosen you for its home. If those things didn't happen, you would probably die.

That's just a cold. What about serious degenerative diseases like osteoporosis or atherosclerosis?

Fair enough. Let's look at osteoporosis first. When our diet and lifestyle causes us to use or lose more calcium than we are consuming, our body compensates by increasing our ability to absorb calcium and decreasing calcium excretion. If calcium loss continues, something must be done to maintain normal blood levels of the mineral. A signal is sent which triggers the production of parathyroid hormone. Parathyroid hormone, in turn, stimulates cells called osteoclasts to increase their activity. Osteoclasts break down some of our bone resulting in the release of calcium into the blood stream to replace the calcium that has been lost.

If this beautifully orchestrated process did not occur, the low blood calcium would lead to increasing malfunction of our muscles, nerves, and other tissues. In other words, for someone whose diet and/or lifestyle causes blood calcium loss, the alternative to osteoporosis is death!

Osteoporosis, therefore, is the result of a wonderful survival mechanism that helps keep us alive during times of famine, ignorance, or stupidity. Most of you reading this are not in a state of famine and the fact that you have chosen my book proves you are certainly not stupid. It is far more likely that you are just ignorant of many of the factors that may cause osteoporosis to be necessary. Beware! After you read my chapter on osteoporosis, the only excuse left will be stupidity because osteoporosis can be prevented, stopped, or reversed in most cases.

OK, now let's look at atherosclerosis, more commonly called coronary heart disease. We will start with an analogy. If you were to spend an entire day raking leaves, chopping weeds, and pruning trees without gloves and you were not used to it, you would probably develop blisters. You would want to protect the damaged skin from further injury so you might put a Band-Aid® on the blisters. Ahh, that feels better, doesn't it?

What happens to people who do those things for a living? Do they spend their entire lives with blisters on their hands? No, of course not. The body is intelligent and builds thicker skin called callus at the points of stress. In effect, the body supplies its own Band-Aid®.

The same thing happens in our arteries. When the artery is irritated over and over by oxidized cholesterol, excess homocysteine, smoking, poor dietary choices, etc. basically two things happen: First the muscular wall of the artery gets thicker at the point of injury and second, a layer of plaque is laid down over the injured site. Just like a callus and a Band-Aid® protects your hand, the thickening and the plaque protects the artery. **The problem is that we keep injuring the arteries over and over again with poor diet and lifestyle choices.** Just as a callus on the hand gets thicker and thicker with repeated stress, the arterial wall thickens and the plaque continues to increase. The space inside the artery is limited and as the crud builds up, blood flow is reduced.

Hey!! I thought you said the body is smart. This sounds pretty stupid to me. The body is killing itself.

Actually it is our lifestyle choices that are stupid. The body makes a survival decision: Is it better to let the irritation eat a hole in the wall of the artery or is it better to put a patch on the area and make it tougher? Which one will lead to the longest period of survival?

Obviously, a hole in the artery would end things pretty quickly. A patch is the intelligent thing to do. Our physiology is very smart. What kills us is repeating our damaging behavior until the stack of Band-Aids® finally blocks the artery. Quoting the famous American philosopher, Forrest Gump: "Stupid is as stupid does".

Dr. Howard Loomis – an enzyme therapy expert - explains it this way: "Disease is an insidious process that begins with small alterations in our body's chemistry. If we don't correct these alterations by changing our diet and lifestyle, the body must compensate biochemically to maintain itself. When our body's ability to compensate becomes exhausted, it must alter physiological function to sustain life. If the process continues, the altered body functions will produce changes in structure."

There are basically three ways to approach this common progression.
1. We can ignore it until it is very difficult to change direction.
2. We can take drugs in an attempt to control our internal chemistry (usually with mixed results).
3. We can provide our body with the internal environment it needs to heal itself.

Eating what our body needs and avoiding the things that produce toxic stress will enhance this healing environment. Obviously the best time to make these changes is before structural damage has occurred. If this nutritional approach is started early enough, the subtle chemical alterations within us are corrected before we are aware there was a problem.

As a chiropractor, I also recognize the importance of optimal communication between the brain, spinal cord, and the rest of the body. It is outside the scope of this book to tell you how chiropractic can enhance this inner conversation, but my experience indicates that it certainly does. I firmly believe that chiropractic should be an integral part of health care.

Chapter 8
A Bone of Contention

We are often told that osteoporosis is caused by not eating enough calcium. Let's look at a couple of studies. Research conducted by Dr. Lawrence Riggs of the Mayo Clinic found that the women with the highest consumption of calcium had just as much bone loss as did those with the lowest consumption of calcium. A more recent Harvard study including tens of thousands of nurses found that those with the highest calcium supplement intake actually had a 45% higher risk of fracture.

Combine that with the knowledge that women in many cultures consume far less calcium than American women yet have very little osteoporosis and it begins to appear that dietary calcium deficiency is not the primary cause.

Quit teasing us, Doc! What the heck is going on here?

There are many factors involved and it would take another book to consider them all, but **the three primary factors are diet, exercise, and hormones**.

Dietary factors

Yes, bones do need calcium **and magnesium, and vitamin C, and vitamin D, and many more nutrients**. This brings us back to the idea of eating a large quantity of a wide variety of vegetables and fruit as well as getting some sunshine regularly.

At least as important as eating the right foods, is avoiding the wrong ones. For example, eating excess animal protein can damage bone in at least four ways.

1. Acid Ash: When animal protein is metabolized, it leaves an acid residue called ash. Our blood, lymph, cerebral spinal fluid, and most of our other body fluids must be slightly alkaline or we will die, so we have several buffering systems to keep the pH of these tissues normal. The most powerful of these buffers is the bicarbonate system. Bicarbonate uses organic sodium (from the plants we eat -- not from table salt). If we don't have enough usable sodium or there is just too much acid, the body goes to the store and gets calcium for the bicarbonate system to use. The calcium store is our bones.

2. Excess Phosphorus: Although our bones need phosphorus, too much in the diet can cause problems in at least two ways. First, phosphorus competes with calcium for absorption so high phosphorus intake can keep the calcium we are eating from getting into our body.   Second, our blood must maintain a proper ratio of calcium to phosphorus. When phosphorus gets too high it stimulates the production of parathyroid hormone. This hormone is the messenger I mentioned earlier that tells those osteoclast workers to break down bone to get more calcium in the blood and bring the ratio back to normal. This keeps us alive, but reduces our bone mass. In addition to meats, dairy products and many soft drinks have more phosphorus than we need.

3. Arachidonic Acid: Arachidonic acid is a type of fatty acid found primarily in animal products. This fatty acid produces substances that promote inflammation, and in excess, can break down bone and inhibit tissue repair. Inflammation is an important part of healing, but when our diet and lifestyle contains too many pro-inflammatory factors and not enough anti-inflammatory ones, we are in trouble. Our bodies can manufacture arachidonic acid when it needs some. Eating it can push us closer to the edge. I believe it was George Bernard Shaw who said, "We dig our graves with our teeth."

4. Homocysteine: Both plant and animal protein provide the essential amino acid methionine, but animal protein has a lot more. Methionine is converted to another amino acid called cysteine. A necessary middle step in this conversion is the formation of a chemical called homocysteine. Excess homocysteine has been implicated in both osteoporosis and coronary heart disease. The body isn't stupid, so it has provided ways to get rid of the homocysteine.

I won't go into the biochemistry of it, but the pathways use vitamin B6, vitamin B12, folic acid, and magnesium to convert the homocysteine back into methionine or into cysteine. When we don't get enough B6, B12, folic acid, and magnesium and/or we overwhelm the system with too much methionine (from a diet with excess animal protein), we are contributing to bone and artery damage.

Other dietary factors that are suspected to increase calcium loss include sugar, caffeine, alcohol, and soft drinks (many contain phosphoric acid, caffeine and sugar – all risk factors).

Exercise

The next major factor is exercise. Bone is a living tissue and responds to physical stress just like muscle – it gets stronger. So any type of exercise that puts more stress than usual on the bones can be helpful. Even gaining weight by eating too much reduces the risk of fracture, but that is not the method I recommend.

A group of women in one study actually gained bone mass simply by jumping up and down 50 times a day. The gravitational stress as you hit the ground and push off again tells your entire body that it needs to become stronger to resist those forces. Jogging, running in place, etc. can also help. If you already have advanced osteoporosis, the force of jumping could actually cause a fracture, so you would need to talk to your doctor about your risk and build up very slowly.

Walking doesn't put as much stress on the bones as the other activities, and recent research indicates that it is not as effective. Walking is, however, a really good way to improve your cardiovascular system, lose weight, control blood sugar, raise HDL (the "good" cholesterol), etc. and is much better for your bones than doing nothing.

Hormones

The third major factor is hormones. Somewhere around age 35, a woman's bone mass begins to decrease at a rate of approximately 1% per year. Then at menopause the decline accelerates to around 3% per year for about 5 years then slows to about 1.5% per year.

John Lee, MD, wondered why bone loss begins around age 35 when estrogen doesn't decline until around age 50. Also, if bone loss is caused by estrogen deficiency, why does Estrogen Replacement Therapy usually just slow bone loss but not reverse it? He came to the conclusion that the medical profession was looking at the wrong hormone.

When a woman ovulates, the ovarian follicle that produces the egg becomes something called the corpus leuteum. This structure produces progesterone. He found that around age 35, women begin to have occasional periods without ovulation. As ovulation decreases, so does progesterone production. Dr. Lee felt that the decreasing progesterone was triggering the bone loss. He found that when his patients used cream that contained progesterone, the progesterone was absorbed through the skin and most of the patients not only quit losing bone, but instead, began to increase their bone density.

To find out how your bones are doing, there are a couple of tests I recommend. The first measures your bone density and is called DEXA (Dual Emission X-ray Absorptiometry). DEXA does not tell you whether you are currently losing, gaining, or maintaining bone. It just tells you the density right now.

You may have lost bone earlier in you life, but now because of lifestyle and dietary changes, the bones may be getting stronger. Or maybe the loss has accelerated. The second test I recommend is a metabolism assay. This test assesses the amount of two chemicals in your urine that indicate how fast or slow bone and/or cartilage is breaking down at the time of the test. The chemicals are pyridenium and deoxypyridenium.

Some women may need estrogen supplementation progesterone, or drugs, but many will do quite well by eating lots of vegetables and fruit, while decreasing or eliminating animal protein, caffeine, sugar and other refined foods, and getting regular weight-bearing exercise. Of course the best time to accentuate the positive and eliminate the negative in your diet and lifestyle is from the very beginning in order to build very strong bones throughout childhood and adolescence. It is not within the scope of this book to discuss non-nutritional approaches. I highly recommend the book **Better Bones, Better Body** by Susan Brown, Ph.D. I have read many books on osteoporosis. Dr. Brown's book is my favorite.

Chapter 9
Nothing to Sneeze At

While driving to work, Jim noticed a little pain in his abdomen. By the time he arrived at his office, the pain had increased considerably. He decided to lie down for a few minutes until the pain went away. It didn't. As the pain became more intense and radiated into his back, Jim began to sweat. After an hour or so, the pain slowly disappeared as mysteriously as it began.

Over the next couple of years, the pain visited often. Sometimes it was only a week or two between episodes, other times it would be two or three months. Jim wondered if it was related to something he was eating so each time it happened, he would think about what he had eaten the day before. He could not make a connection.

One day, the pain just wouldn't go away and Jim decided to go an emergency room. Blood work indicated the possibility of gall bladder inflammation. A sonogram was performed. The gall bladder looked fine, but the bile duct leading from the gall bladder to the small intestine was swollen. A surgeon recommended removing the gall bladder the following morning. Jim said that didn't make sense to him because the gall bladder looked OK. The surgeon assured Jim that "If we jerk that thing out of there in the morning, you'll never have this pain again." Jim refused. The pain had subsided, so he went home.

Whoa Doc! This is supposed to be a chapter on allergy -- not gall bladder disease. Maybe you have a brain allergy.

Well, I understand what you're saying, but trust me and read a little more. Here is where the story gets really interesting. A couple of days later, Jim was introduced to a book by Dr. James Breneman, a medical doctor specializing in allergies. He said that gall bladder symptoms were usually caused by food allergies. I was – oops, I mean Jim – was skeptical. OK, OK. The story is about me. I was skeptical because I know how most of us think. To a carpenter, everything looks like a nail. So I figured to this allergist, everything looks like an allergy. Besides, I wasn't sneezing, I was hurting. But Dr. Breneman had evidence.

He said that symptoms disappeared in <u>all</u> of his gall bladder patients when the offending food was identified and eliminated from the diet, even when the organ was full of stones. When the food was re-introduced, the pain would return. He said the allergic reaction causes the bile duct to swell, which restricts the flow just as if a stone were blocking the duct. So when a patient tells a doctor about the pain and diagnostic imaging finds a bag full of stones, the doctor assumes that the stones are the cause of the pain. If there had been stones in my gall bladder, I might have had surgery. It seems logical, but according to Dr. Breneman's work, it may be quite wrong.

Dr. Breneman listed the foods that most often caused problems for his patients. For some people, onions were the problem. Others reacted to chocolate. The doctor developed a list of a number of foods that caused problems and put them in order of the frequency of involvement. The food that triggered "attacks" in more people than any other was eggs. I didn't eat eggs very often, but I did remember that my wife had prepared some eggs two or three days before I went to the emergency room. I eliminated eggs from my diet and never had another pain – until I was at a nutrition conference in Florida a couple of years later.

I was enjoying a luxurious buffet and noticed some key lime pie on the dessert table. I had never tasted key lime pie so I had a slice. It was delicious and since I was unlikely to eat it again in Texas, I had another slice. This was on a Saturday. On the following Tuesday, the pain hit. You might think it was a psychological connection, but I didn't know key lime pie had eggs in it. Unwittingly, I had performed a classic challenge test – a reintroduction of the suspected allergen.

It was a double-blind experiment. At the time of the test, neither the researcher (me) nor the subject (me again) knew the food contained eggs.

That was a long story, but it brought out two very important points: 1. The symptoms did not occur until two to three days after the exposure, and 2. I had abdominal pain instead of the "typical" allergy symptoms. Let's talk about both of these things.

Most of us are familiar with the "usual" allergies. The dogwood tree spits out pollen and within a very short time, we begin to sneeze, wheeze, itch, etc. We also know of people who are allergic to strawberries or peanuts or some other food. Almost immediately after eating it, they have the above symptoms or worse. These immediate reactions to foods are usually pretty easy to identify. The problem is with "delayed" allergies. I had eaten six to eight meals with a total of a couple of dozen different foods between the time I ate the eggs and the onset of symptoms. I may have never figured it out if I hadn't seen Dr. Breneman's book.

Delayed allergies involve a component of the immune system called Immunoglobulin G (IgG). The IgG binds with the offending substance to form what is called an immune complex. The immune complexes circulate through the blood stream and then are deposited in some organ or tissue of the body. In some people, the target tissue might be the bile duct, in others it could be the joints (arthritis), brain (lack of concentration, irritability, etc.), muscles (muscle pain, fatigue), or just about anything else. So you can see that allergy can appear in many disguises. In many cases, the patient and the doctor never even consider that the symptoms may be allergy related.

What determines the location where these circulating immune complexes will be deposited? The mechanism is far too complicated for you to understand. (That's doctor talk for "I don't know"). But it probably has something to do with genetic predisposition. We may inherit a genetic tendency for a particular malady, but those genes don't have to express themselves. Modifying genetic expression is a very hot topic right now among enlightened, intelligent, talented, handsome nutritionists such as myself.

All right, Dr. Wonderful, don't get carried away. So if the allergy might show up as anything and it may be days after the exposure, how can I know if an allergy is involved and what I'm allergic to?

I'm going to ignore your sarcasm and terrible sentence structure. There are two basic ways to find out.

The first is called an "elimination diet". You eliminate the most likely allergenic foods from your diet for about three weeks to see if it makes you feel better. Then you add the suspect foods back into your diet -- one new food every third day -- to see which one(s) cause a reaction. This method has the advantage of being inexpensive and it can identify foods that you are sensitive to, but not truly allergic. For example, if drinking milk causes bloating and diarrhea, it is probably due to a lack of the enzyme lactase – not an allergy. The disadvantage is being difficult to complete because it is restrictive. This method may also miss some foods that are not allergenic to most people, but are to you.

The second method of identifying a delayed allergy is laboratory testing. Until recently, the available allergy tests were effective only in identifying the IgE or immediate allergies. Tests have recently been developed for IgG or delayed reactions. The best labs test for both IgE and IgG and even include sub-sets of IgG. Most of the laboratories have food panels, inhalant panels, chemical panels, etc.

While not perfect, these tests are effective at pinpointing most allergens, but have the disadvantage of being expensive. This expense is relative, however. People who have spent thousands of dollars trying to get rid of their migraines, irritable bowel, fatigue, joint pain, asthma, etc. might consider a few hundred dollars to identify and correct the underlying problem as being pretty cheap.

An allergy test would not find the milk/lactase problem mentioned above, but an elimination diet would. A nutrition-oriented health care professional can help you decide what is best for you and provide you with the details.

Chapter 10
Is There A Doctor in the Joint?

I picked up a big book on nutrition the other day and read the introduction. This was a book by a well-known doctor and endorsed by a well-known hospital. Among other things, the book said that anyone who says arthritis can be helped by changing the diet is a quack. Usually comments like that just roll off me like water off a duck's back, but this time it really ruffled my feathers!

This doctor has apparently not kept up with the scientific literature. For example, in volume 338, pages 899 to 902 of the medical journal *Lancet*, there is strong evidence that diet does make a difference. For example, two matched groups of arthritis patients were taken to a health spa. One group ate their normal diet – probably a little better because the spa staff was preparing it. This was the control group. The other group was put on a diet containing no gluten and no animal products. This was the experimental group.

After four weeks, the control group reported that the pain had decreased a little. The improvement was probably due to better food preparation and the relaxing atmosphere of the spa. Laboratory work, however, made it clear that the disease was continuing to progress.

The vegetarian group not only had significantly less pain, and less joint stiffness, but several other markers had improved as well. Objective things like the number of swollen joints, Erythrocyte Sedimentation Rate – a measure of inflammation – grip strength, and white blood cell count improved in the vegetarian group, but not in the control group.

A personal example: A patient came to see me with red, swollen joints in her hands from rheumatoid arthritis and was actually crying from pain. She wanted to know if I could do anything to help. I told her that there was nothing I could do, but plenty *she* could do. I told her to immediately stop eating meat, eggs, and dairy products, and to take a tablespoon or two of flaxseed oil every day. She came back in three days later with no redness, no swelling, and no pain. She said that she hadn't felt that good in years. Diet does make a difference for many people and it isn't difficult to explain why.

Why did you tell your patient to stop eating meat, eggs, and dairy products?

The main reason is that those foods contain a significant amount of arachidonic acid. You may recall from the chapter on fats and oils, that arachidonic acid is a direct precursor to inflammation. Inflammation is a necessary part of healing, but when we eat lots of the wrong things, we put ourselves into a pro-inflammatory state. This means that inflammation caused by acute or chronic conditions may get so bad and last so long that it interferes with healing instead of being a part of it.

In addition to increasing inflammation, arachidonic acid increases osteoclast activity. Osteoclasts are the cells that break down bone. Arachidonic acid also stimulates the production of collagenase – an enzyme than breaks down cartilage. A loss of bone and cartilage and an increase of inflammation and pain sounds a lot like arthritis to me.

It gets worse. Arachidonic acid also can increase swelling by making the blood vessels more permeable, and it inhibits proteoglycan production. Proteoglycan is structural material our bodies use to repair damage to bone and cartilage. So eating the wrong things can increase the damage to cartilage and bone, increase pain and swelling, and at the same time, inhibit natural repair. Diet does make a difference.

Note: By "meat" I mean all animal flesh. Some patients don't have a problem with poultry, but some are very sensitive to it. To be on the safe side, I have them stay off all animal stuff, at least for a while.

Does a person with rheumatoid arthritis have to give up those foods forever?

Probably not. I normally ask patients to follow a totally vegan diet for three weeks. It rarely takes longer than that for symptoms to dramatically decrease. Then the patient can carefully and slowly add other foods into their diet. They should only add back one new food every third day to see if they react to it. Even if they can now tolerate some of these foods, I recommend that they eat them very sparingly if at all. If avoiding the foods made the symptoms go away, eating them again may ultimately result in the pain and tissue destruction they were experiencing before. And before you add cow milk back into your diet, please read my chapter titled *Dairy Dilemma*.

Now you are probably wondering why I recommended the flaxseed oil. Again, think back to the chapter on fats and oils. Flaxseed is rich in the omega-3 fatty acid alpha-linolenic acid. Omega-3 fats tend to produce anti-inflammatory chemicals so excessive inflammation will be reduced. We eat far fewer of the anti-inflammatory foods than we used to. My recommendations to my patient were designed to correct the imbalance and get things back to normal as soon as possible. After the inflammation was gone, I was able to provide chiropractic care to improve joint function and further improve her ability to heal.

See? Once you understand the basics, this stuff isn't that hard to figure out. You just restore balance by removing things that interfere with good health and increasing the things that enhance it.

Many arthritis patients are also sensitive to a class of plants called "nightshade" plants. Nightshades include tomatoes, white – not sweet – potatoes, eggplant, and peppers such as bell peppers and chili peppers. Tobacco is also a nightshade plant, but most of us don't eat tobacco. I guess a lot of cowboys and baseball players do, but most of us don't.

Here is another puzzle for you. Lots of people eat meat and eggs, and drink milk. Many develop arthritis but some don't. Why not? The main reason some are "attacked" is that they probably have a genetic predisposition to that condition. If the irritants are removed, however, even those who are genetically predisposed often get better.

Research also suggests it may be strongly related to "leaky gut". You may recall from the chapter **Gut Reaction**, that when the intestines are inflamed, undigested proteins make it through the wall into the blood stream. Antibodies attack these foreign substances and while they're at it, attack our own bone joints and muscle that are similar to the tissue we ate. Many of the medications prescribed for arthritis patients help stop the pain, but increase the intestinal damage. Some of them also inhibit joint repair. Fixing the digestive system is often the key to stopping this condition.

There are several approaches to this including the previously mentioned "4R" program, enzyme therapy, elimination diet, anti-inflammatory flavonoids in ginger, turmeric, and other plants, depending on the patient's biochemically individual needs.

How are those individual needs determined?

Well, the long answer would be to talk about all the possible lab tests, exam findings, environmental factors, social situation, etc. combined with my years of training and experience. The short answer is that you may need to see a knowledgeable professional to fine-tune your program. **Remember that this book provides general information, not protocol for an individual patient. A professional should evaluate any serious condition.**

Another form of arthritis, even more common than rheumatoid arthritis, is osteoarthritis. This type is often thought of as being a normal result of aging and the "wear and tear" of life. But often a person will have one arthritic knee or hip while the other one – in most cases, the same age as the bad joint – is doing just fine. In fact one of the hallmarks of identifying osteoarthritis by x-ray is that it is asymmetrical – only on one side. More recent research indicates that it may be due to improper biomechanics brought about by minor injury and/or muscle weakness or imbalance. One study seems to support the idea that weakness or imbalance of the quadriceps muscles is one of the main causes of osteoarthritis.

As the cartilage breaks down, people often take ibuprofen or other non-steroidal anti-inflammatory drugs to relieve the pain. These drugs do suppress pain, but also can suppress the body's ability to produce the building blocks for repair.

The most common non-drug approach is to take supplements of glucosamine sulfate, chondroitin sulfate, or a combination of both. Research indicates that glucosamine sulfate is not as effective for pain as ibuprofen for the first couple of weeks, but sometime around the third week, it actually becomes more effective. It also has the advantage of being one of those building blocks so it enhances healing instead of inhibiting it. A study of people with arthritic hips found that taking 1500 milligrams of glucosamine sulfate for a year resulted in the joint space actually increasing back towards normal.

Other forms of glucosamine are less expensive, but most of the research I have seen used glucosamine sulfate. At the time of this writing, it is the form I recommend. However, I am always willing to change my mind as new research and clinical experience comes along. Chondroitin sulfate is also found naturally in cartilage. The molecules are much larger than glucosamine molecules and some feel much harder to absorb. Others believe that adding it to the glucosamine works better than glucosamine alone. Again, research and experience will settle the question over time.

Chapter 11
The Heart of the Matter

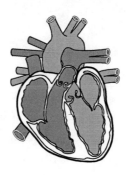

I'm sure you know that more men die from heart disease than any other cause. Are you also aware that more women die from heart disease than any other cause? When I ask people to name the disease that kills more women, most say, "breast cancer". **The truth is, heart disease kills twice as many women as all cancers combined.** In fact, about half of us will die from some form of heart disease.

Let's look at some research and ask some questions. Maybe we can figure out how to change these numbers.

Mark Hyman, M.D. says, "Heart disease is not one disease. It is a label we ascribe to the final product of multiple metabolic and genetic variations that give rise to atherosclerosis." Let me put this another way. Is heart disease caused by genetics? High cholesterol? Low HDL? High triglycerides? Saturated fat? Hydrogenated fat? Insufficient vegetables and fruit? Not enough exercise? High homocysteine? Low folic acid? Smoking? Sugar? Enzyme deficiency? Low magnesium? Low vitamin E? High iron? Diabetes…? The answer is yes.

Of course each of those answers raises more questions: How can a person lower their genetic risk? How can we lower our cholesterol (or homocysteine, etc.)? The good news is that a few simple things have profound effects on these risk factors. Exercise, for example, can lower total cholesterol, raise HDL, lower blood sugar and risk of diabetes, strengthen the heart muscle, build collateral arteries, increase oxygen uptake, lower blood pressure, and much more. We will look at other things at the end of this chapter.

Before I show you how to dramatically lower your risk of heart disease, let's look at some very interesting research findings.

Here is the research I mentioned earlier. In 1982 the *Journal of the American Medical Association* published a study that tested the effect of polyunsaturated oil on heart disease. Previous studies had proven that these oils lower cholesterol. It was expected that this would therefore lower the risk of heart attack. In this study, two groups were put on a low-fat diet. In addition to the diet, the people in one of the groups consumed four tablespoons of corn oil – a common source of polyunsaturated oil. As expected, the corn oil group had lower cholesterol. But surprisingly the corn oil group also had twice as many heart attacks than the other group.

Why? What the heck is going on here? Corn oil is supposed to be good for us and cholesterol went down – but heart attacks went up.

I don't know the answer for sure, but I'll bet my theory will hold water (or oil). Go read the chapter ***Fries, Lies, and Heart Attacks*** again, then you can probably figure it out too.

Are you back? Did you read it again? OK, a little quiz: What are the three things that can damage dietary oils? You are absolutely right! Light, heat, and oxygen damage them. I'm willing to bet that the corn oil these people got was the same stuff that we buy at the grocery store. Before it ever gets in the bottle, it is exposed to lots of heat, light and oxygen and even more light after it is bottled. Even if the experimental group didn't cook with the oil, it was already damaged.

Now here is the second quiz question: What do the light, heat, and oxygen produce in the oil? Right again! Free radicals. So these people were gulping oil that had been oxidized by processing. The oil lowered their cholesterol, but the free radicals damaged their arteries leading to more heart attacks. That's my theory and I'm sticking to it just like plaque sticks to damaged arteries.

Another study followed the experience of a group of Jews who moved from Yemen to Israel. Consumption of animal fat did not change much. Consumption of sugar, margarine, and vegetable oil increased significantly. Their coronary artery disease increased dramatically. OK. Your last quiz question is an essay question. Why did these people experience more heart disease? Uhuh – yes – right. Wow! You are absolutely correct. See how smart you are? It's the same as in the corn oil study. And the increase in sugar and margarine consumption probably increased levels of triglycerides and trans-fats, which also may have increase their risk.

Here is a bonus question. Isn't this a great book? Just this one piece of information can extend your life and save thousands of dollars. And the book is full of great information. What a wonderful investment you have made. Tell your friends about it. ☺

Before we talk about other risk factors and how we might prevent heart disease, you might like to know how to assess your risk. Typically you get blood work done that shows your cholesterol (including LDL, HDL, etc.) and triglycerides. Collectively these are known as your blood lipids. If your doctor reports that your blood lipids are normal, you feel relieved. **Did you know that almost half of all people who have heart attacks have normal blood lipids?** That's right. Our usual method of screening for heart disease risk misses half the people who have a problem. By the way, the very first symptom of heart disease that many people experience is death, so it might be a good idea to do a better job of assessing risk.

Here are six additional blood factors that are very helpful. I'll keep this as brief and non-technical as possible.

1. Homocysteine: Research has shown that people with the highest 25% of homocysteine levels have triple the heart attack risk compared to the people with the lowest 25%. This is independent of cholesterol levels

Homocysteine is an intermediate by-product of our metabolism of an essential amino acid called methionine.

When everything is working properly, the methionine converts to homocysteine, then the homocysteine converts to harmless chemicals or back to methionine. This important conversion requires three cofactors: Vitamin B_6, Vitamin B_{12}, and folic acid. When we don't have enough of those nutrients, or we are eating too much methionine, homocysteine can build up and damage arteries – and bone.

We already talked homocysteine in the osteoporosis chapter. As you recall, animal protein has more methionine than does plant protein. So too much meat and dairy along with not enough plants in our diet can be a contributing factor for too much homocysteine and therefore, heart disease.

2. Lipoprotein (a): An accurate marker for clogging of the carotid arteries in your neck and probably the best indicator of risk for cerebral infarction (stroke).

3. Apolipoprotein A-1: The primary protein in HDL (the "good" cholesterol) so in general, higher is better. Low Apo A-1 level is a good predictor of early heart attack in young men.

4. Apolipoprotein B: The primary protein in LDL (the "bad" cholesterol) so in general, lower is better. The ratio of Apo B / Apo A-1 is probably the best predictor of early coronary artery disease in children and young adults.

5. C-Reactive Protein: This has been widely used as a marker of inflammation. It has been recently discovered that people with elevated C-Reactive Protein have triple the risk of heart attack and double the risk of stroke.

Inflammation from any source should be considered an independent risk factor for cardiovascular disease.

6. Fibrinogen: Significantly increases blood coagulation and is increased by inflammation. Fibrinogen also promotes atherosclerotic plaquing, clot formation, and thickening of the blood. Smoking, obesity, oral contraceptives, sedentary lifestyle, diabetes, hypertension, inflammation, and stress can increase fibrinogen. Fibrinogen is decreased by exercise, control of blood sugar, essential fatty acids, stress management, quitting smoking, and weight reduction.

Some medical laboratories may not be set up to test for all these additional factors, and most doctors do not order them routinely. Some laboratories, such as Great Smokies Diagnostic Laboratories in Asheville, North Carolina put them all together along with the blood lipids in a Comprehensive Cardiovascular Risk Assessment. If you or your doctor would like more information, they can be reached at www.gsdl.com

OK. Now that we have covered some ways to find out whether or not we are at risk, let's look at some more factors that influence our heart health.

Sugar: It is estimated that the average person in 1750 consumed 6-8 pounds of sugar per year. In 1950 it was 120 pounds per person per year. And now in the beginning of the new millennium, it is 170 pounds per person per year.

So? Other than cavities – which dentistry is controlling – what's wrong with sugar? I love the stuff.

Good question. Here are a few of the research findings about sugar.

Sugar consumption can increase triglycerides, platelet aggregation (increasing the risk of blood clots), uric acid (associated with gout), blood pressure, and total cholesterol. It decreases the helpful HDL.

Research conducted by Dr. William B. Grant at NASA Langley Research Center uncovered several interesting considerations:

> **1. Sugar appears to be the most important dietary heart risk factor in women.**
>
> 2. The likely mechanism is that it raises serum triglycerides and very low-density lipoprotein levels.
>
> 3. Sugar intake may account for over 150,000 premature deaths per year from heart disease in the U.S.
>
> *Orthomolecular Medicine, 1998*

Coffee: Here is a quote from a recent study.
> "After adjustments were made for age, systolic blood pressure, total cholesterol, triglycerides, diabetes, alcohol use, and the physical activity index, men who consumed 24 ounces of coffee

per day experienced twice the risk of stroke as compared to nondrinkers."

Fats and Oils: Even thought there is a separate chapter on this topic, it is worthwhile to focus in on how these fats relate to heart disease. First, most of us eat lots of hydrogenated or partially hydrogenated oils. Almost all commercial baked goods and processed foods have lots of them. During hydrogenation, up to 60% of the normal molecules are converted to trans-fats. As mentioned before, trans-fats block essential fatty acid function. Hogs fed trans-fats had more extensive aortic deposits than those fed beef tallow or butter. In my opinion, hydrogenated fats are <u>very</u> bad for you.

You already know that heat damages oils. Research tells us that eating heated corn oil creates more damaged arteries than when the oil is not heated and the damage from heated oil is even more extensive if the oil is also exposed to oxygen. Every time a basket of French fries are dropped into a vat of hot oil, oxygen is being mixed into the oil.

Two types of oil appear to be good for the heart and I'll bet you know what they are. Olive oil has been shown to lower LDL, raise HDL, and decrease lipid peroxidation. Omega 3 oils such as found in green leafy vegetables, flaxseed, and fish will decrease clotting and lower triglycerides. Of course when the omega 3 oils are heated, damage is the result.

Plants: One study said that eating two raw carrots each day can lower cholesterol by 10-20%. Chemicals in plants called phytosterols and saponins can decrease cholesterol absorption from a meal by up to 64%. Garlic and onion decrease LDL, VLDL, and platelet aggregation (the tendency to clot) while increasing HDL and fibrinolysis. One study indicates that ginger is as effective as aspirin at decreasing platelet aggregation.

Exercise: The Harvard Physicians Health Study found that exercising once or twice per week decreased the risk of heart attack by 36%. Exercising three or four times a week produced a 38% decrease in risk – only a little better than once or twice. But exercising five or six times a week decreased the risk by 46%. This tells us that **even a little exercise can decrease our risk of a heart attack by more than a third and if we make a habit of doing it almost every day, our risk is reduced by almost half.** For this study, exercise was defined as simply any activity vigorous enough to work up a sweat.

There are many nutrients that have been shown to decrease our risk, but it is way outside the scope of this chapter to discuss them all. Nutrients such as magnesium, vitamin C, taurine, niacin, vitamin E, chromium, selenium, and others have been scientifically shown to be helpful. So do we need to buy 30 bottles of supplements to get all of this? Not at all. We need to eat lots more vegetables, fruit, and other whole foods.

A study of the effect of diet on high blood pressure found that only 2% of vegetarians had high blood pressure compared to 26% of matched non-vegetarians. The best foods to help lower blood pressure include celery, garlic, onions, nuts, seeds, green leafy vegetables, and foods with omega 3 fatty acids.

Celery? I thought that stuff just had a little fiber and water.

That's what a lot of people think, but research has found all vegetables and fruit contain lots of phytochemicals that we didn't know about. Celery contains something called 3-n-butyl phthalate, which lowers blood pressure. Animal studies demonstrate a 12-14% decrease with the equivalent of 4 stalks per day. One man who tried this method dropped his blood pressure from 158/96 to 118/82 in just one week by eating ¼ pound of celery per day. That's just 4 ounces!

That sure seems worth trying when a study published in the *Journal of the American Medical Association* found that beta-blockers – commonly prescribed for high blood pressure – only help about 1/3 of the patients who take them. The side effects of beta-blockers include fatigue, sexual problems, nightmares, poor exercise tolerance, decreased circulation and more.

There may be cases where drugs are needed, but I feel that dietary changes, exercise, stress management, and a healthy lifestyle should be the first line of defense.

Chapter 12
Good Cells Gone Bad

When you hear about cancer prevention, it usually involves mammograms, prostate exams, blood tests, etc. Please understand that these have absolutely nothing to do with prevention. They are methods of early detection. Detecting a problem early may be a good thing, but not nearly as good as preventing it in the first place.

I'm going to approach this chapter a little differently. Research has provided a great deal of information about the causes and prevention of cancer that most people seem to be unaware of. I'm going to give you bits of studies along with where they were published.

Most of the studies speak for themselves, but I'll add a note here and there when I think it might be helpful. Any underlining, bold type, etc. is mine. I will cover prostate cancer in some detail, but the same things that are associated with prostate cancer are also associated with many other types of cancer. Then I will cover a few of the things that are unique to other cancers. Methods of treatment will change as we learn more, but the principles of prevention seem to be quite stable.

PROSTATE CANCER

"…the effectiveness of prostate cancer early detection remains a dilemma, since **no randomized, controlled study has ever demonstrated disease-specific mortality reduction from any test or procedure**…"

"Cost-effectiveness calculations of prostate cancer early detection have not been possible due to **the lack of any data demonstrating reduction in mortality from any test or procedure...**"
CA 1993; 43:134-149

Autopsies reveal prostate cancer in 70% of men over 80 and in 30-50% of men over 50 who have died from unrelated causes. *The Prostate 1990; 16:187-197*

NOTE: *This means that most men, if they live long enough, get prostate cancer. It also tells us that it usually doesn't kill them. In fact, they often don't ever know they have it. If cancer is detected early by PSA (Prostate Specific Antigen), many doctors recommend a "watchful waiting" approach. If it is an aggressive form of cancer, something may need to be done. But the best thing is to do everything possible to prevent the disease from developing in the first place.*

Black men living in Africa have a low rate of prostate cancer. <u>Migration to the United States increases the risk ten-fold.</u>
U.S. Public Health Service, Disease Prevention/Health Promotion: The Facts 1997

NOTE: *This strongly suggests that the primary factors are diet, lifestyle and other environmental exposures – not genetics.*

Among black men in the United States, those eating frequent portions of pork, beef and eggs had an almost threefold increased risk of prostate cancer. Those with frequent consumption of carrots, spinach, collards, and poultry had a significantly decreased risk. For both black and white men in the study, high consumption of fat was the major dietary risk factor.

Journal of the NCI 1987;78(5):869-874

In a study of 8,000 men of Japanese ancestry, the risk of prostate cancer increased substantially when these men moved to Western society. Eating large amounts of butter, cheese, eggs, and margarine increased the risk. Maintaining the traditional Japanese diet (rice, tofu, vegetables) kept the risk low.

Cancer Research 1989;49:1857-1860

Another Japanese study indicates that low intake of fresh fruits and vegetables doubled the risk of prostate cancer.

The Prostate 1988;12:179-190

A United States study found that the consumption of meat, fish and all forms of animal fat was associated with an increased risk of prostate cancer.

Journal of the NCI 1983;70(4):687-692

In a study of 14,000 Seventh-day Adventist men, those eating a higher amount of meat products <u>and particularly fish</u>, had an increased risk of prostate cancer. The men who had been raised vegetarian had a 25% lower risk of prostate cancer than the men who had adopted that lifestyle later in life.

Cancer 1989;64:605-612

NOTE: *We are told that the oil in fish is good for our hearts, but this study indicated that eating fish increased the risk of prostate cancer. Maybe there is something about fish we haven't learned yet, or maybe the increase is from the toxins the fish have picked up from polluted waters. In any case, there appears to be a problem.*

Seventh-day Adventist men who are lacto-ovo vegetarians have a 70% lower risk of prostate cancer mortality compared to the general male population of California.

Cancer Research 1975;35:3513-3522

A 21-year prospective study of 6,700 Adventist men revealed a dose-related increase in prostate cancer mortality and the consumption of milk, cheese, eggs, meat, and poultry.

Am J Epidemiology 1984;120(2):244-250

NOTE: *The Seventh-day Adventist population is often studied because most of them live a healthy lifestyle and about half of them are vegetarian (mostly lacto-ovo meaning they do consume dairy products and eggs). This makes it easier to determine the effects of diet. Notice that even with dairy and eggs, the men have 70% lower risk of dying from prostate cancer than those who also eat animal flesh (beef, pork, poultry, fish, etc.). And among those lacto-ovo vegetarians, those who eat the least dairy and eggs have the lowest risk.*

There is a strong association between elevated testosterone and prolactin and prostate cancer. Increased saturated fat consumption and obesity is associated with increased testosterone and prolactin.

Am J Clinical Nutrition 1985;42:127-134
Am J Clinical Nutrition 1990;51:371-377

In 1975, a study by Armstrong and Doll concluded that the consumption of animal fat is the leading risk factor for prostate cancer mortality. Subsequent research seems to support their conclusion.

International J Cancer 1975;15:617-631

"Dairy products consistently have been associated with an increased risk of prostate cancer..." "One study...found that calcium consumption, which can lower circulating 1, 25 dihydroxyvitamin D (1, 25 D), was associated with higher risk of advanced prostate cancer..."

"RESULTS: Calcium intake was an independent predictor of prostate cancer."

Cancer Causes Control 1998;Dec(6):559-556

Another study found a significant dose-related risk between milk consumption and prostate cancer. Compared to those drinking no milk, the relative risk was 1.2 for those drinking 1 glass of milk a day. The relative risk was 5.0 for those drinking 2 or more glasses a day. That means drinking only 2 glasses of milk each day increased the risk of prostate cancer 500%.

Oncology 1991;48(5):406-410

"For Prostate cancer, epidemiologic studies consistently show a positive association with high consumption of milk, dairy products, and meats."
Adv Exp Med Biol 1999;472:29-42

"The incidence of prostate cancer in Greece could be reduced by about two-fifths if the population increased the consumption of tomatoes and reduced the intake of dairy products, and substituted olive oil for other added lipids."
Eur J Cancer Prev 2000 Apr;9(2):119-123

"Overweight men had a significantly higher risk of fatal prostate cancer than men near their desirable weight."
"Suggestive positive associations were also seen between fatal prostate cancer and the consumption of milk, cheese, eggs, and meat."
Am J Epidemiol 1984 Aug;120(2):244-250

"Biomarkers, including testosterone and insulin-like growth factor, and nutritional factors, especially meat, fat, and dairy intake, have been linked to greater risk of disease."
"Higher consumption of selenium and vitamin E, fructose/fruits, and tomatoes all have been associated with reduced occurrence of prostate cancer..."
Semin Cancer Biol 1998 Aug;8(4):263-273

How is dairy consumption believed to be associated with prostate cancer?

The above study mentions that insulin-like growth factor has been linked to prostate cancer. Milk contains bovine insulin-like growth factor that is identical to human insulin-like growth factor. It appears to be a risk factor and drinking skim milk doesn't help. It's still in there. The purpose of high amounts of growth factor in milk (cow, human, etc.) is to help the baby grow rapidly up to the time of weaning. We are not designed to handle the consumption of this powerful hormone throughout our lives.

You may have heard of supplements designed to increase the amount of insulin-like growth factor in your body. The ads say that the amount of growth hormone decreases as we get older so if we take it, our youthfulness will be restored. I believe those supplements are bad for you for the same reason it's bad to consume it in milk. I do not recommend those supplements.

NOTE: *I know there is a lot of repetition here. That is intended. I want you to see that there is a great deal of research in many different scientific journals over several decades saying the same thing. I'm sure you have already heard that eating more vegetables and fruit and less animal stuff is good for you – but did you know the evidence was this clear and this strong and this important? I didn't, until I started digging into the journals. Our evening news tells us all about the latest drug that's supposed to help us with weight control, allergies, depression, etc., but they usually don't tell us about this.*

OK. We have talked a lot about prostate cancer. Let's take a look at some of the research on other forms of cancer.

BREAST CANCER

Genetics is believed to account for only 10-15% of breast cancer cases. The environment, including nutrition, is thought to play a significant role in predisposing women to this cancer. Asian women eating their traditional diets have a low incidence of breast cancer, but second generation emigrants to the United States lose this protection.

Am J Clin Nutr 2000 June: 1705S-1707S

According to the Harvard Nurses Study, the following things increase the risk of getting breast cancer: Oral contraceptives, Hormone replacement therapy, Two or more alcoholic drinks per day. Women with low vitamin A intake and increased monounsaturated fat intake (as in olive oil) had a lower risk.

American Journal of Nursing June, 1996

A study pooling the data from more than 40 previous studies involving more than 60,000 women found that taking estrogen replacement therapy more than doubled the risk of getting breast cancer.

Imperial Cancer Research Fund - Oxford

Many breast tumors are estrogen-driven. The amount of estrogen produced is associated with the amount of fat in the diet. On high fat diets, more estrogen breaks free from its carrier molecules and becomes biologically active. Vegans (who eat no animal products at all) have significantly lower estrogen levels than non-vegetarians.

JNCI 1987;78(4)
JNCI 1987;79(6):1225-1229
Am J Cl Nutr 1988;48:787-790

OTHER CANCERS

Dr. Daniel Cramer of Harvard University found that women with ovarian cancer consumed significantly more dairy products – especially yogurt – than women without ovarian cancer. The apparent mechanism is that the consumption of dairy exceeds the capacity to break down galactose. (Note: Refer to the Dairy chapter to learn more about galactose.)

Lancet 1989;2:66-71

A seven year study of 35,156 women, ages 55 to 69, found that those who consumed more than 36 servings of red meat a month doubled their risk of developing non-Hodgkins lymphoma compared to those eating less than 22 servings per month.

Journal of the American Medical Association

The Harvard Nurses Study of 88,410 women has found that a higher intake of fruits and vegetables is associated with a lower risk of non-Hodgkin's lymphoma. Vegetables demonstrated stronger protection than fruit. Higher intake of cruciferous vegetables was also associated with decreased risk.

Dept. of Nutrition, Harvard School of Public Health
Cancer Epidemiol Biomarkers Prev 2000 May;9(5):477-485

Lung cancer patients show a history of high consumption of saturated fat. Lung cancer is less likely among those with high intake of green vegetables (other than lettuce) and more likely among those with a high intake of whole milk.

J Nat Cancer Inst 85:1906 Dec, 1993

Cancer in the colon, breast, prostate and pancreas may be caused by heterocyclic amines formed during the broiling of frying of fish and meats. Cell proliferation and development of preneoplastic and neoplastic cells involves oxidation reactions. Health promoting nutrition involves the daily intake of five to ten vegetables and fruits.
Food Chem Toxicol 1999;39(9-10):943-948

NOTE: *Recently it has been discovered that these carcinogenic chemicals are formed in animal flesh no matter how it is cooked – even when boiled.*

"...even moderate intake (of alcohol) appears to increase cancers of the breast and large bowel."

"Higher intake of meat and dairy products has been associated with greater risk of prostate cancer."

"Higher intake of vegetables and fruits has been associated with lower risks of many cancers."
Dept. Epidemiology, Harvard School of Public Health

Natural killer cells seek out and destroy cancer cells. Vegetarians have more than twice the natural killer cell activity found in non-vegetarians.
Nutr Cancer 1989;6:705-710

Smoking has a strong association with colon cancer after a 30-year latent period. Current use of **oral contraceptives** increases the risk of breast cancer, coronary heart disease, and stroke. **Moderate alcohol use** increases the risk of breast cancer and benign polyps in the colon. **Red meat** intake increases the risk of colon polyps and cancer.

Harvard Nurses Study

OK, I think you've gotten the picture. We actually know quite a bit about what to do and what not to do to significantly reduce our risk of getting cancer. Some of you might be interested in just how fruit and vegetables help prevent cancer. There are probably several mechanisms.

First of all, if we fill ourselves with vegetables, we will have less room in our stomachs for the dead animal parts that appear to be related to some cancers.

Secondly, there are thousands of chemicals in plants called phytochemicals (See the chapter titled *Plant Power*). We are a long way from even identifying all the chemicals, much less understanding what they do, but what we have learned so far is very encouraging.

Normal cells reproduce when they need to and stop when they need to. For example when you cut yourself, new cells will grow to close the wound. As the healing progresses, a signal causes the cells to stop growing. Cancer cells don't stop growing when they are supposed to. Fruits and vegetables contain chemicals that help us maintain normal cell function and growth while inhibiting pre-cancerous and cancerous cell proliferation.

Third, the chemicals in these plants actually increase the ability of your immune system to search out and destroy these deadly cells. One type of cell involved in protecting you is the natural killer cell. You read in the research above that vegetarians have more than double the natural killer cell activity compared to non-vegetarians.

Fourth, the vegetables and fruit provide vitamins, minerals, carotenoids, flavonoids, and thousands of unpronounceable chemicals that improve the health and function of every cell, tissue, and organ of your body.

Simply put, there is absolutely nothing more important in the prevention of cancer than eating lots of good, fresh, whole foods and minimizing your exposure to those things which are harmful. **Do it.**

Chapter 13
The Dairy Dilemma

I grew up associating milk with nurturing, love, cookies, grandma, good health, strong bones, good teeth, etc. One of my uncles was a dairy farmer. I loved spending time with my cousins working with the cows and crops, and drinking lots of fresh, cold, raw milk. There was also plenty of homemade butter and wonderful ice cream actually made with fresh cream. Wow!

Many, many years later, while living and practicing in a small New Mexico community, I read an interesting article in the local newspaper. The president of the New Mexico Farm and Livestock Bureau was criticizing a group called the **Physician's Committee for Responsible Medicine (PCRM)** for expressing some health concerns about milk.

I had never heard of the Physician's Committee for Responsible Medicine and had no idea what they had against milk, but the article made me curious. I tracked down the organization and asked for information. What I received started me on a very interesting journey.

The first item I read was a paper published by the **American Academy of Pediatrics** in the medical journal *Pediatrics* in 1992. The paper provided the following information:

Cow milk causes gastrointestinal blood loss in a large proportion of infants leading to iron deficiency. Some infants can lose large quantities of blood.

"The composition of cow's milk...may decrease the bioavailability of iron from other dietary sources such as infant cereals."

"...iron deficiency in early childhood may lead to long term changes in behavior that may not be reversed even with iron supplements sufficient to correct the anemia."

"Whole cow's milk feeding would narrow the margin of safety in situations that may lead to dehydration." This is due to the high sodium content of milk.

"Infants fed whole cow's milk have low intakes of iron, linoleic acid, and vitamin E, and excessive intakes of sodium, potassium, and protein."

"The American Academy of Pediatrics recommends that whole cow's milk and low iron formulas not be used during the first year of life."

Have you heard any of this before? Did you know that feeding cow's milk to infants could cause them to bleed internally? And this isn't from some radical group. It's from the American Academy of Pediatrics.

That's just the tip of the ice cream -- I mean iceberg. As I researched more deeply, I found that there were some epidemiological studies (studies of large populations) that found an association between milk and Type 1 diabetes. The studies found that as the consumption of milk increased, so did the risk of Type 1 diabetes. The research also indicated that the risk increased as the prevalence of breast-feeding decreased.

Of course there could be other factors involved. The way science normally investigates a finding like this is to perform animal studies and then, if warranted, human studies. That's exactly what was done in this case. There is a strain of laboratory rats that are predisposed to diabetes. In fact about 50% of them usually become diabetic. A study published in July 1992 in the *New England Journal of Medicine* found:

"Diabetes does not occur in diabetes-prone rodents reared on a diet free of cow's milk for the first two to three months of life, indicating that cow's milk proteins can trigger the disease."

OK, but we aren't rats. We are peoples. What does it have to do with us?

You are right. The epidemiological and animal studies strengthen the evidence, but can be misleading. We must look at humans to find out if humans are really affected. One study discovered that all of the diabetic children in the study had antibodies to a cow milk protein called Bovine Serum Albumin (BSA). This is an immune response. It means that 100% of these diabetic children had produced an army of antibodies to attempt do destroy the invading BSA in the same way that the body defends against a bacteria or virus.

As research continued, the Bovine Serum Albumin was examined more closely. That led to the discovery that the BSA contains a chain of amino acids (called ABBOS) which is identical to proteins on the insulin producing cells of the pancreas. **So when the antibodies go to war against the milk protein, they also go to war against the proteins on the pancreas.** The antibodies can't tell the difference between the ABBOS in the cow milk and the pancreatic cells because there is no difference. They are identical.

Now we have epidemiological evidence, animal evidence, and human evidence that there is a connection between milk consumption and one form of diabetes – and we have a mechanism.

There are research articles from the U.S., Finland, Spain, Germany, Switzerland, England, and elsewhere that show concern. Here are quotes from two abstracts:

"The results suggest that young age at introduction of dairy products and high milk consumption during childhood increase the levels of cow's milk antibodies and that high IgA antibodies to cow's milk formula are independently associated with increased risk of IDDM (Insulin Dependent Diabetes Mellitus)"
Diabetologia, 1994

"RESULTS – The introduction of cow's milk-based formula into the diet before 3 months of age was associated with an increased risk. High dietary intake of cow's milk protein in the 12 months before the onset of diabetic symptoms was also associated with an increased risk."
Diabetes Care, 1994

There are many more studies from several countries I could quote, but I think you get the idea.

If drinking milk causes diabetes, why don't I have it?

It appears that there must be both a genetic predisposition plus a trigger for the disease to manifest. A study published in the journal *Diabetes* in 1993 was able to divide subjects into high and low risk groups based on a molecular marker (HLA-DQB1). If you don't have the genetics, the trigger won't cause the disease. If you do have the genetics, but don't consume the trigger, you won't get the disease. It takes both. The studies suggest that there may be a few other triggers in addition to cow milk protein including nitrites, nitrosamine compounds and fetal viral infections. The primary trigger, however, seems to be in the cow milk.

The American Academy of Pediatrics reviewed the research and selected about 20 studies that met stringent scientific standards. Quoting from their paper published in *Pediatrics* on November 5, 1994:

> "This analysis concluded that there was a modest, but statistically significant association...between the early introduction of cow's milk (and/or early termination of breast-feeding) and the development of IDDM in childhood"

**NOTE: IDDM means Insulin Dependent Diabetes Mellitus.

All of this research talked about *early* introduction of cow's milk. When asked if it was safe for children to start drinking cow milk *after* infancy, Michael Klapper, MD said, "I wouldn't bet my son's pancreas on it."

Theoretically all food should be completely digested into its basic components before being absorbed through the gut lining. For example, protein should be reduced to individual amino acids before being absorbed.

It is believed that for the first three or four months of life, the gut is excessively permeable or "leaky". Large molecules of incompletely digested food can pass through the intestinal wall and into the blood stream. Our immune system then produces antibodies to fight against these large molecules, so **when babies are fed cooked grains or other hard-to-digest foods too early, they may develop allergies to those foods.** It was believed that after the first three or four months, there is "gut closure" and now large protein molecules won't leak through the intestinal wall. Apparently, this belief was unfounded.

In a study of intestinal permeability, scientists chose Bovine Serum Albumin (BSA) as their test substance because its molecules are quite large and should not pass into the bloodstream intact. The BSA was fed to healthy young adults. A significant amount was absorbed intact into the blood stream. If Bovine Serum Albumin can be absorbed intact into the bloodstream of adults, consumption of cow's milk may still be a risk factor for genetically predisposed children even if exposure is delayed until well past infancy.

OTHER CONSIDERATIONS

If you are already an adult, you probably won't get Type I diabetes from dairy products, but you might want to look at some other research. A Spanish medical journal reported that consumption of milk and cheese was constantly positively correlated with pancreatic cancer mortality rates in men. Egg consumption showed the highest cancer correlation in women, while eating fruit helped protect against the cancer in both men and women.

Most of you have heard of lactose intolerance. Some people stop producing the enzyme lactase and when they drink milk, the undigested lactose can ferment causing gas, bloating and discomfort. Lactose – milk sugar – is made of two other sugars, glucose and galactose. Some people digest the lactose just fine, but can't break down the galactose. According to a study reported in the *Journal of Nutrition* in August of 1993,

> "Milk ingestion was dose-related with cataract risk in lactose digesters (particularly in diabetics) but not in lactose maldigesters".

This means that in some people who digest the lactose with no problem, drinking milk may increase the risk of cataracts. The more milk they consumed, the higher the risk. The researchers believe this is due to a build up of galactose. <u>There are no symptoms to warn us.</u> A Harvard Medical School study published in the *Lancet* found that the galactose problem might also be associated with increased risk of ovarian cancer.

HEART DISEASE

Here is another potential risk. Two researchers – Kurt Oster, MD and Donald Ross, Ph.D. – discovered that an enzyme called xanthine oxidase (X-O) may be causing heart damage. They say that X-O destroys an important component of muscle tissue called plasmologen. A small amount of X-O is produced in the liver, but not much is found in healthy tissue, but an article in the *Proceedings of the Society for Experimental Biology and Medicine* reports that diseased arteries contain biologically active X-O. A possible source is bovine milk xanthine oxidase (BMXO).

An epidemiological study of 13 countries found increased heart disease to be directly associated with increased consumption of homogenized milk. Another double-blind study discovered that **as homogenized milk consumption increased, so did the BMXO antibodies in the blood.** This indicates that the xanthine oxidase in the homogenized milk produced an immune response against it.

What does homogenization have to do with it? Fat is normally absorbed into the lymphatic system, not directly into the blood stream. The liver then destroys the BMXO before it gets into general circulation. Homogenization, however, breaks the fat into such small particles that the fat is absorbed directly into the blood stream, carrying the BMXO with it, and possibly increasing the risk for heart disease.

AUTISM AND SCHIZOPHRENIA

Research at the University of Florida suggests a possible connection between autism, schizophrenia, and a protein found in cow milk. Animal studies indicate that the inability to break down a milk protein results in the production of a compound called beta-casomorphin-7. When this chemical reaches areas of the brain known to be involved in autism and schizophrenia, it causes the brain cells to dysfunction.

In human research it was found that 95% of the autistic and schizophrenic children studied had 100 times the normal amount of the milk protein in their blood and urine. **When these children were put on a milk-free diet, at least 80% of them no longer had symptoms of autism or schizophrenia.** The primary researcher – Dr. J. Robert Cade – said, "We now have proof positive that these proteins are getting into the blood and proof positive they're getting into areas of the brain involved with the symptoms of autism and schizophrenia".

INSULIN-LIKE GROWTH FACTOR 1 (IGF-1)

Here are some studies to consider:
1. The more IGF-1 there is in a man's blood, the higher his risk of prostate cancer.

J Nat Cancer Inst 1998;90:876-9

2. The Harvard Physicians Health Study found that IGF-1 concentrations are strongly linked to prostate cancer.

Science 1998;279:563-6

3. Serum IGF-1 has been found to be higher in women with breast cancer than in women without breast cancer.
Lancet 1998;351:1393-6

That's interesting, but what does this have to do with cow milk?

4. Cow milk contains pre-formed insulin-like growth factor that is identical to human IGF-1
Science1990;249:875-84

5. A study involving older adults found that the addition of three 8-oz servings per day of non-fat or 1% milk for 12 weeks caused a 10% increase in IGF-1 levels
J Am Dietetic Assoc 1999;99:1228-33

6. An earlier study showed similar results in adolescent girls.
British Medical Journal 1997;315:1255-60

7. A review of the scientific literature found that cancer risk paralleled milk consumption in numerous studies.
Am Inst for Cancer Res 1997 p.461

Do you realize the significance of all this? The top medical research journals are telling us that for many people, cow milk is likely linked to gastrointestinal problems, type 1 diabetes, some cancers, heart disease, cataracts, autism, schizophrenia, and much more that I haven't mentioned here.

The bottom line is that fresh, raw, whole cow's milk is a wonderful food – for baby cows.

Chapter 14
Going Against the Grain

OK, it's time for a major confession – My name is Jim and I'm a carboholic. I crave carbs. More specifically, I crave bread, cake, cookies, tortillas, crackers, granola, shredded wheat, etc. More accurately, I am a <u>recovering</u> carboholic and I no longer crave these things. I assure you, however, that if I had just a little of any of the above items, the cravings would come roaring back. I would want more, more, more.

Here is another confession. This chapter is being written after I thought the book was finished. But I must tell you how I got the doughnut off my back. Allow me to share my personal experience.

I'm sure you are aware that sometimes there is a difference between knowing the right thing to do and being able to do it. And sometimes what we think we know can use a little fine-tuning. I knew I should not eat refined carbs from candy, pastries, etc. but they seemed to have some sort of hold on me. If someone brought a couple dozen homemade cookies or some other delight, I would tell myself to leave them alone. But sooner or later, the internal cookie monster would take over and I would lose the battle – and one was rarely (never) enough.

My mom was heavy. Her parents were heavy. Most of her siblings are heavy, so I come by my gravitational challenge honestly. I could talk to you about genetics, lipoprotein lipase (LPL), set point theory, etc., but my rather extensive knowledge of these factors didn't help me lose weight and so probably wouldn't help you either.

I tried eating less. I tried to avoid the bad stuff. I tried high carbohydrate, low fat programs with no meat and lots of pasta and veggies. I even tried high protein, low carbohydrate programs. Nothing seemed to help for more than a short time. The main saboteur of all these attempts was strong cravings. I could eat a nice salad, stuff myself with spaghetti marinara – and lots of garlic bread – and still want something more.

I would arrive home with my stomach still uncomfortably full and eat a bowl of cereal. I know it sounds stupid and it isn't something easy to admit, but the cravings would become overwhelming. I've never been addicted to a drug, but I'm sure it's not much different. It seemed my body was missing something very important and forcing me to try to find it.

Then a few weeks ago, my wife forwarded an email to my office. It was about a nutrition lecture that she thought I would like to attend. She was right. A few days later, I was listening to Dr. Douglas Graham. Dr. Graham is an energetic, well-muscled, athletic man. The reason I mention it is because for the last 25 years, he has eaten nothing but raw fruit, vegetables, nuts and seeds – mostly fruit.

Dr. Graham said lots of interesting things that night, but I paid special attention to what he said about cravings. He said that craving starch or other sugars means you haven't eaten enough fruit. He recommends nothing but fruit for breakfast and lunch. Then for dinner, he says to eat more fruit, then a nice salad with perhaps some avocado and nuts to add a little fat. Grains and grain products are totally eliminated.

That sounded pretty extreme, but the guy looked extremely healthy. Perhaps extreme health requires extreme action. The scientist in me was curious and open enough to give his ideas a try, although I felt fairly confident that I would not be able to stick to it more than a day or two. After all, who would want to live without bread? I bought a couple of Dr. Graham's books and went home.

Within two days, my life-long cravings were gone. A few days later, my wife had to remind me that it was time for dinner. For the first time I can remember, I had forgotten about it. Also I have always used lots of salt. I salted watermelon, cantaloupe, and almost everything else I ate. My need for adding salt to my food is gone.

After a few days, I tried an experiment. I was a little hungry in the middle of the afternoon. Instead of having a piece of fruit, I had a peanut butter sandwich on some really good sprouted whole grain bread. An hour after eating the sandwich, I was hungrier than I had been before I ate it. It was about half way through the next day before the cravings and the hunger calmed down again. As I said, I'm a recovering carboholic. And as I'm learning, maybe I'm more of a grain-oholic.

At the meeting, Dr. Graham's associate, Professor Rozalind Gruben – who has eaten nothing but raw plants for the last 15 years – said that some grains contain at least 15 different opiate compounds. Wow, I say. No wonder

I'm addicted to the stuff. Maybe that's why we consider bread as a "comfort" food. What really amazed me is that in all the years I have studied nutrition and in the hundreds of books I've read, that little piece of the puzzle slipped past me.

First of all, I wondered if it was true. I have learned not to accept much without some investigation. I turned to the all knowing Internet. A web search turned up some very interesting information.

In **The Dairy Dilemma**, I told you about something in milk called beta-casomorphin-7 that – according to Dr. Robert Cade – is likely associated with autism and schizophrenia. This chemical is an opiate or opioid. In fact the word casomorphin is derived from casein – a milk protein – and morphine. These chemicals are called opioids because they trigger the same receptors and have similar actions as opium.

Gluten – a protein found in many grains including wheat, oats, barley, rye and triticale – also contains opioids called gluteomorphins or gliadinomorphins. (Oat gluten may not contain morphins.) These opioids are very similar to casomorphins and may have similar effects.

In addition to the grains themselves, products made from the grains may also contain gluten. These products include malt, grain starches, hydrolyzed vegetable proteins, textured vegetable proteins, grain vinegars, soy sauce, grain alcohol, flavorings and the binders and fillers found in some vitamins and medications.

Paul Shattock, a researcher at the University of Sunderland in England, has written articles suggesting that the opioids in gluten may have the same relationship to autism as the opioids in milk. To learn more about this, check out www.autismndi.com

So according to what I've learned from Dr. Graham, my cravings were probably due to two things: An attraction (addiction?) to the gliadinomorphins in the grains and a need for simple sugars to fuel my cells. Fruit provides enough sugar to satisfy, but also enough dietary fiber to keep it from adversely effecting insulin production. And at least for me, it wipes out the need for the morphins.

The most surprising aspect is how easy it has been so far. A recent potluck lunch at work provided an abundance of cakes, cookies, and other morphin-laden goodies and **not only was I not tempted, I truly did not want them in my body**. My office is near our break room. Previously I could hear these items calling my name, but now they are strangely silent.

Even though I have not followed the program perfectly – I have had a few cooked meals – the pounds are melting away while I'm feeding my cells what they really need. The key for me seems to be lots of fruit and absolutely no grain. I have not yet had enough experience with this to recommend it to everyone, but anything that provides lots of whole, fresh, ripe, raw, organic fruits, vegetables, nuts, and seeds is a step in the right direction. Genetic analysis indicates that 90,000,000 Americans may have some degree of gluten sensitivity that can be related to arthritis, cancer, ear infections, and much more. See the book "Dangerous Grains" in the Recommended Resources.

Section 3

Putting It All Together

Chapter 14
Plant Power

As I write this, "phytochemical" is the current buzzword. Science is catching up with Mom. Phyto simply means "plant." So phytochemical (phytonutrient) is just the fancy name for the things in plants that our bodies utilize. Mom said, "Eat your fruits and vegetables." Now the American Cancer Society, National Cancer Institute, American Heart Association, National Institutes of Health, and many others are saying the same thing. The research is overwhelming: People who eat diets rich in a variety of fresh fruits and vegetables are healthier than those who don't.

It has taken a while for researchers to get the big picture and there is still some confusion. We have a tendency to look for the "active ingredient" in a food instead of seeing the food as a synergistic blend of thousands of active ingredients. For example, it has been observed that populations that eat lots of foods rich in beta-carotene have less lung cancer. So researchers gave groups of smokers beta-carotene supplements and compared them to smokers not taking the supplements. Much to their surprise, the supplemented smokers got lung cancer more often than those not taking the pills did. Why?

Research has now shown that giving a high dose of isolated beta-carotene can actually suppress the activity of other anti-oxidants. Foods rich in beta-carotene are also rich in zillions (approximately) of other important nutrients that work together. There are thousands of other phytonutrients that have been identified and probably thousands more that we don't even know about. Our bodies work best using food -- not bits and pieces isolated from food.

Another characteristic of phytonutrients is specificity. We've known for a long time that vitamin C is water-soluble and does much of its work in the watery tissues of the body. Vitamin E is fat soluble and helps fight oxidation of cell membranes and other fatty tissues.

It gets even more specific than that. Lycopene (found in tomatoes, watermelon, strawberries) is especially adept at protecting the prostate and the skin. Lutein (found in spinach and other green, leafy vegetables) protects the macula of the eye. The macula is the focal point on the retina. Macular degeneration is the leading cause of blindness in the elderly.

Now that science has discovered plants, many researchers are trying to isolate the active ingredients and make "nutriceuticals." But if we take a beta-carotene supplement, we miss out on alpha-carotene and the 600 or so other carotenoids. If we take a lycopene supplement, we don't get the lutein, zeaxanthin, quercitin, hesperidin, etc., etc., etc. If we take sulforophane (a protector against cancer found in broccoli, cabbage, and others) we miss the powerful health-sustaining effects of indole carbinols (found in the same vegetables). What we need is a wide variety of fresh foods that contain <u>all</u> these wonderful nutrients.

Unfortunately, most foods we get at the grocery store aren't as fresh as they could be. Many fruits and vegetables are picked days or weeks before ripeness so they won't be over-ripe by the time they make it to the store. Many of the important nutrients and enzymes are concentrated in the food during the ripening process. If the food is taken off the vine before this occurs, much of the nutrition is lost.

Even if we do have fresh fruits and vegetables available, we don't eat nearly enough of them. We don't eat sufficient quantity, quality, or variety. Surveys indicate that most Americans eat from a group of about 18 different foods. We eat those same foods over and over again. Some cultures eat about 100 different foods regularly. In Japan, the number one recommendation for good health is to eat at least 30 different foods every day.

It's easy to add variety to your diet. Explore the produce section of your market and try new things. If you live in a metropolitan area, go to Asian markets, European markets, Middle-Eastern markets, etc. You are likely to find some great new nutritious foods. The same applies to grains and fruit. Try kamut, quinoa (pronounced keen-wah), spelt, amaranth, papaya, mango, kiwi, star fruit, and more.

We need to eat as many fresh fruits and vegetables as possible, but most of us don't. Some of us just don't like them. Others have trouble digesting some of them.

Diabetics and dieters often shy away from fruit and especially fruit juices because of the higher sugar content.

Helping people change their eating habits is one of the most difficult things to do in my practice. Those who make the change often see amazing results. Unfortunately, many people just can't or won't do it. I found something to help those people. It is a food-based supplement called Juice Plus+®. This product is a combination of 17 fruits, vegetables and grains, so it has many of phytonutrients we have been talking about, delivered in a convenient form.

The foods are picked ripe and very carefully processed using state-of-the-art technology. The resulting product is basically concentrated food.

Can you really get much nutrition in those little capsules?

I was skeptical about this myself. But research at several universities around the world indicate that it increases blood levels of antioxidants, lowers free radical damage, significantly improves the immune system and helps protect DNA, and much more.

The concept behind the product makes sense and the research backs it up. I take it myself and recommend it to others.

Chapter 15
A Simple Plan

The simplest way to implement these principles is to eat a plant-based diet. But, when I talk about vegetarianism with my students, there is usually one who says that every vegetarian he has met looks weak and sick. Several of his classmates agree. And I agree that some people who say they are vegetarian don't look very well. However there are a couple of things we need to think about.

One possibility is that the person has been sick for a long time and has just recently turned to a vegetarian diet in attempt to become healthier. Maybe the diet hasn't had time to work yet.

Possibility number two is that they are eating a very unhealthy version of a vegetarian diet. Donuts are vegetarian along with white bread, over-cooked vegetables, candy bars, partially hydrogenated oils, and much more trash.

Number three is that their definition of "vegetarian" is different from what you have in mind. There are many types of vegetarian diets. For example, the most common form is lacto-ovo vegetarianism. These folks eat no animal flesh, but do consume milk and eggs. There are also vegans, who eat no animal products of any kind. Some vegetarians follow a macrobiotic path while others eat only raw foods. Some eat primarily fruit and others seem to think that fish is a vegetable – they are called pescovegetarians. When the word "vegetarian" is used here, it means lacto-ovo vegetarian, because that is what the vast majority of vegetarians choose. For example, about half of Seventh-day Adventists eat meat and about half of them are vegetarian. Of the vegetarian half, about 98% of them are lacto-ovo vegetarians.

To be fair, we must consider a fourth possibility as to why some vegetarians look sickly. Maybe vegetarianism is just plain unhealthy. Lets look at some research.

1. Non-vegetarian Seventh-day Adventist men have up to three times more heart disease than the vegetarian Adventists. Vegans have a lower risk than the lacto-ovo vegetarians.

Prev Med 1984;13:490-500

2. Lacto-ovo vegetarians have cholesterol 14% lower than omnivores (who include animal flesh in their diet), and vegans have cholesterol 35% lower than omnivores.

J Am Diet Assoc 1991;91:447-453

3. Subjects who ate a 30% fat diet including lean meat lowered their cholesterol by only half of the reduction achieved by subjects who ate a lacto-ovo vegetarian diet.

Am J Clin Nutr 1989;50:280-287

4. The level of trans fatty acids in the subcutaneous fat of lacto-ovo vegetarians is about 1/3 lower than in non-vegetarians. No trans fatty acids were found in the subcutaneous fat in vegans who ate no refined products.

Am J Clin Nutr 1988l48:920

5. Arachidonic acid (found primarily in animal products) leads to series 2 eicosanoids, which constrict arteries and increase platelet aggregation.
Am J Clin Nutr 1990;52:1-28

6. The prevalence of blood pressure higher than 160/95 was 13 times higher in the non-vegetarians in this study.
Am J Clin Nutr 1983;37:755-762

7. A study of more than 6,000 people found that the cancer mortality rate among vegetarians for all cancers combined was only half that of the general population.
Br Med J 1994;308:1367-1371

8. Consumption of animal products just 1.5-3 times a week increased the risk of breast cancer compared to eating it less than once a week
Jpn J Cancer Res 1994;85:572-577

9. Men who consumed high amounts of dairy products had a 70% increased risk of prostate cancer. Those who also took calcium supplements had about a 300% increased risk.
Harvard – Health Professionals Follow-up Study

What! Calcium supplements increased the risk of prostate cancer?

I have absolutely no idea why that happened. But once again, it shows us the wisdom of sticking to whole foods and being careful about separating nutrients from their synergistic plant-mates and getting things out of balance.

10. A large study of Seventh-day Adventists indicates that the combined effect of eating meat, eggs, milk, and cheese increased breast cancer risk by 3.5 times.

J Clin Nutr 1988;48:739-748

We could continue with tons of research about how vegetarians have stronger bones, less bladder cancer, reduced abnormal cell proliferation, lower bile acid production, and on and on, but I think you have gotten the idea by now. In general, vegetarians are healthier that flesh eaters. Vegans are even healthier.

Here is one more study, then I'll finish up the chapter with some great quotes.

A study at Georgetown University put one group of Type II diabetics on the diet recommended by the American Diabetes Association and put another group on a vegan diet. After three months, the subjects on the vegan diet had a 59% greater decrease in fasting blood sugar than those on the ADA diet and needed less medication. The vegans also lost twice as much weight, and experienced a greater decrease in cholesterol levels.

Dr. William Castelli – the director of the well-respected Framingham heart study – said this: *"Some people scoff at vegetarians, but they have a fraction of our heart attack rate and they have only 40% of our cancer rate. On the average, they outlive other men by about six years."*

Albert Einstein – pretty much the smartest guy around (he is still around, relatively speaking) – *"Nothing will benefit human health and increase the chances for survival of life on earth as much as the evolution to a vegetarian diet."*

My favorite comes form Dr. Dean Ornish: *"Eating a vegetarian diet, walking ever day, and meditating is considered radical. Allowing someone to slice your chest open and graft your leg veins to your heart is considered normal and conservative."*

Sometimes us human beans are very strange indeed.

Epilogue

Well, there you have it. I hope you experienced an "Aha!" or two and maybe even "Eureka!". Please understand that the chapters on specific conditions were written to give you some ideas about how to prevent these diseases, not treat them. For that, you need to see a health care professional.

This book is incomplete. There is far more information out there and new research is published every day. I want to tell you about enzymes and about nutrition for children. We could also talk more about different types of diets, about the implications of alcohol consumption and many other topics. Maybe those topics will be covered in another book. My goal was to keep this one short and simple.

The astute reader will have noticed that the basic principles of good nutrition apply to everyone. The exact same foods that help a person stay healthy will also nourish the bodies of those who are ill. And it is so simple if we will **just do it**.

1. Eat <u>lots</u> of fresh vegetables and fruit – **be sure the majority of it is raw.**

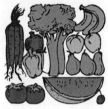

2. Eliminate refined and processed foods (even if they come from the health food store, made from organic ingredients)

3. Minimize or eliminate animal flesh, animal fat and animal secretions (dairy)

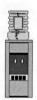

4. Drink plenty of good water

5. Don't do drugs (including alcohol, nicotine, and caffeine)

6. Exercise a little every day

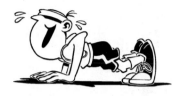

Those six simple steps are the essence of this entire book. I had to write more, of course, because you wouldn't have paid me for a book with just one page. Even more important, you now know why each of those steps is so important to your health.

You don't have to change everything at once. Every step in the right direction takes you closer to good health. When you make each change, make it totally. Don't tease your taste buds. Your taste will usually adapt within two to three weeks. Make a commitment to stick with any healthy change – without cheating – for three weeks. Three weeks is a lot shorter than forever. You can do it. At the end of the three weeks, decide whether or not you want to continue for another three weeks. Figure out what needs to be added, eliminated, or adapted.

If you do these things, you will likely be amazed at the changes you experience.

W. Clement Stone said, *"Big doors swing on small hinges"*. Small changes can make big differences if you do them completely. And once you get the hang of it, you might try some bigger hinges and swing some huge doors.

It really isn't difficult to be healthier. Yes, you may have genetic limitations. But you have far greater control of the expression of those genes than you may imagine (read **Genetic Nutritioneering** by Jeffrey Bland, Ph.D. and **Turn Off the Fat Genes** by Neal Barnard).

I truly hope these words have been meaningful and enjoyable to you. As the healthy changes accumulate, you will learn more about what works best for you. I wish you the very best life has to offer. Remember that health is not just a matter of chance – it is also a matter of choice.

I shall tell you a great secret, my friend. Do not wait for the last judgment; it takes place every day.
                                                Albert Camus

You have the power.
The choice is yours.

Choose Extreme Health.

Recommended Resources

The list below includes some reader-friendly and informative books that I have enjoyed.

Better Bones, Better Body – Susan Brown, Ph.D.
This is by far my favorite book covering osteoporosis and hormonal changes related to aging. Dr. Brown's intelligence and experience as a medical anthropologist brings a fascinating and useful perspective to this topic.

Dangerous Grains–James Braly, M.D., Ron Hoggan, M.A.
The subtitle says it all: *Why Gluten Cereal Grains May Be Hazardous to Your Health.* This sounds strange because grains are the foundation of the food pyramid. We are constantly being told that whole grains are good for us. In fact, many of the books in this section recommend eating lots of whole grains. This book, however, says that for some people, grain consumption creates serious problems. Before you say "hogwash", read this book. It is controversial, important, and fascinating.

Digestive Wellness–Elizabeth Lipski, CCN
Learn more about this extremely important subject. This book will make the learning fun. Ms. Lispki not only tells us how our digestive system works, but provides excellent information on how to make it work better.

Excitotoxins–The Taste That Kills–Russell Blaylock, MD
Have you wondered how MSG, aspartame, and other chemicals really affect our bodies? Dr. Blaylock is a board certified medical neurologist who will give you all the

information you need. This is the most technical of the books on this list, but well worth the effort.

Fast Food Nation – Eric Schlosser
If you read this book, you will never again visit a fast food restaurant without thinking about what you have learned. Mr. Schlosser covers not only the food, but also the tremendous impact this industry has had on our economy and culture.

Food for Life – Neal Barnard, MD
Neal Barnard is the founder and president of the Physician's Committee for Responsible Medicine (PCRM). The book covers healthy eating principles based on PCRM's New Four Food Groups – The Whole-Grain group, The Vegetable group, The Fruit group, and the Legumes group. Menus and recipes are included.

Genetic Nutritioneering – Jeffrey Bland Ph.D.
People with a family history of breast cancer, heart disease, diabetes, etc. have no reason to feel doomed. Just because we have a genetic predisposition for a disease doesn't mean we have to get the disease. Dr. Bland, a nutritional biochemist, discusses the antecedents, triggers, and cofactors that must also be present for these genes to be switched on. If we embrace the good and avoid the bad, our chances for a long and healthy life are greatly increased.

Heal Your Heart – Kitty Gurkin Rosati
Kitty Rosati is the Nutrition Director of the Duke University Rice Diet Program. This program was developed over 50 years ago by Dr. Walter Kempner and has helped thousands of people. The program may seem

somewhat extreme, but I would remind you that extremism in the defense of health is no vice (those of you old enough will recognize who I am paraphrasing).

Mad Cowboy – Howard Lyman

Mr. Lyman is a fourth-generation Montana dairy farmer and cattle rancher who ran a feedlot operation for 20 years. He knows cattle. Oprah's interview with him led to both of them being sued by a group of Texas cattlemen for "food disparagement". Did you know that you can get sued for saying something bad about food? That's just the beginning of what you will learn in this fascinating book. It is full of well-documented information that I wasn't aware of even after years of study in the field of nutrition. If nothing else, I think you have to admire Mr. Lyman's courage. By the way, the changes in his life have resulted in his losing 130 pounds and lowering his cholesterol by more than 150 points. Whether you agree or disagree with him, his book is worth reading.

The McDougal Program – John McDougal, MD

When Dr. McDougal was a company doctor on a pineapple plantation in Hawaii, he noticed that among the Asians, the older workers were healthier than the younger ones. He learned that the primary difference was diet. This book provides a program that saves lives. Wait until you read what happened to Sam Waterman in only 12 days. Wow!

Mega Health – Marc Sorenson, EdD

This is one of my favorites. This book covers the same basic principles as many of the others listed here, but it combines easy reading with an amazing number of scientific references. The chapters cover diet, exercise, heart disease, cancer, diabetes, arthritis and much more. It is an excellent read and an excellent reference.

The New Fit or Fat – Covert Bailey, PhD

This is a fun, easy-to-read small book that is stuffed with great information. He covers the basics of good nutrition and exercise in a very entertaining way. His earlier version is just called *Fit or Fat*. Be sure you get the new updated version.

No More Ritalin – Mary Ann Block, DO

After a difficult medical experience involving her own daughter, Mary Ann Block decided to become a physician. If you would like to learn more about her drugless approach to Attention Deficit Disorder and associated conditions, then you will benefit from this book.

Nutripoints – Roy Vartabedian, PhD

We know that apples are good for us and refined sugar can be bad, so how about apple pie, that has both? Dr. Vartabedian developed a point system for analyzing food that accounts for both its good and bad components. His system includes a book which explains the program and lists the nutripoints for thousands of foods, video and audio tapes to help you get started, and a chart listing some of the highest point foods on one side and the lowest point foods on the other. This is a logical, easy approach to eating better.

The Raw Secrets – Frederic Patenaude

As I mentioned in the book, I am currently experimenting with a grain-free raw diet. In the process, I have read several books on the topic and have learned from them all. The one that seems most practical and realistic to me is this one. The subtitle – The Raw Vegan Diet in the Real World – sums it up nicely. If you are interested in giving this a try, you need to read this book. It can be ordered at www.rawvegan.com. Another good resource for raw food information is Dr. Douglas Graham at www.doctorgraham.cc

Reversing Heart Disease – Dean Ornish, MD

Dr. Ornish conducted the first scientific study proving heart disease can be reversed by lifestyle changes. The story of this study and its dramatic results are told in this interesting book. The study compared two groups. One ate a low-fat vegetarian diet, meditated, and practiced yoga. The other followed the guidelines of the American Heart Association.

The Road to Immunity – Kenneth Bock, MD

In these toxic times, the immune system is extremely important. Dr. Bock tells how it works and how to make it stronger in this very accessible book.

Turn Off the Fat Genes – Neal Barnard, MD

While being genetically predisposed to carrying more fat presents unique challenges, it is possible to overcome them. Using the same principles that Dr. Bland outlines in his *Genetic Nutritioneering*, Dr. Barnard zeros in on the fat genes, showing us how to inhibit their expression. This is great information.

Contact Information

If you are interested in ordering more copies of this book, they can be ordered from my website: www.drguest.com

If you have any comments about the book, you can email me at: drguest@drguest.com

I will not be able to respond to all emails due to time constraints, but your comments are appreciated. I will respond to all that I can. I will not diagnose or make specific recommendations via email. A health care professional should be consulted regarding your specific situation.